SAVING FACE

WITHOUT LOSING YOUR MIND

Bringing Mindfulness to Your Cosmetic Procedure

ALAN GOODWIN, Ph.D.

Saving Face Without Losing Your Mind

Printed in the United States of America
ISBN Imprint: Mind Thrive Media
Hardcover ISBN: 979-8-9866495-0-4
Paperback ISBN: 979-8-9866495-1-1
Ebook ISBN: 979-8-9866495-2-8

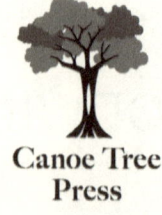

Canoe Tree
Press
4697 Main Street
Manchester Center, VT 05255
Canoe Tree Press is a division of DartFrog Books

TABLE OF CONTENTS

ACKNOWLEDGEMENTS

Writing this book involved a journey that began years ago when I saw my first client who was considering undergoing a cosmetic procedure. No list of sources of help and motivation to write this book would be complete without noting the role my clients have played.

I feel very lucky to do work that I love. Every day, people entrust me with very private information. They rely on me to help them find their way through profoundly challenging periods. What a gift that is. The work is difficult, but it is also tremendously rewarding. I am continually growing and evolving, driven to refine and improve my clinical methods. The ultimate source of this motivation is the connection I feel to the people I serve. And so, to anyone I have counseled, thank you. You are integral to the joy I feel as I begin each and every psychotherapy session and you have played a central role in my writing this book.

For many years, I knew what I wanted to say on this subject but I struggled to find an effective way to say it. I had been accustomed to very different kinds of writing. Breaking free of styles that were appropriate for legal briefs or psychological journals required instruction, practice, and a lot of time.

Ultimately, my dedication was rewarded when I turned my draft over to a wonderfully skilled editor named Molly Winter. With Molly's help, this book truly came to life. I also feel so grateful to have had the help and guidance of Gordon McClellan and the folks at Canoe Tree press. They have been enormously helpful with a range of aspects related to publication.

I want to express special appreciation to Mr. Jamie Keenan. Mr. Keenan is the brilliant cover artist who, somehow, was able to turn a concept into what became a strikingly beautiful and evocative front cover. There is absolutely no doubt that the front cover could never have emerged without his patience, dedication, and mastery.

During the years I devoted to writing and re-writing this book, I had many occasions to be reminded of how grateful I feel to be surrounded by an extraordinary group of friends, colleagues, and family members. Yolanda Noack and Carolyn Okazaki are both exceptionally insightful psychotherapists who are also dear friends. Their moral support and reflections were invaluable in more ways than I can say. There are so many other friends who offered encouragement along the way. To Chris, Lisa, Edna, Corinne and so many others: thank you. Your support breathed new life into my process more times than I can count.

Marshall Zweig is another friend whose tireless assistance is difficult to quantify. Some days he played the role of an editor, on many days he wore his well-fitting marketing guru hat, and on still other days he served as a consultant regarding cover design. Regardless of the day, his friendship, intelligence, artistic sensibility, insane knowledge base, passion, and compassion made an invaluable contribution.

I especially want to note the role my family has played. Well into my third decade of providing psychotherapy, every day I am reminded of how lucky I was to have been born into a family full of love and humor. I know that my parents' unconditional love and support will always live within me and will fuel everything I do. What a gift to have that awareness. Equally important, the love and support of my three sisters, Denise, Stacie, and Andrea, is ever-present and continually nurtures my growth.

CHAPTER 1

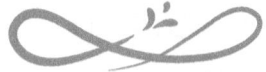

Beginning the Journey

A journey of a thousand miles begins with a single step.

— Laozi

Getting Started

"I've always thought the whole idea of cosmetic surgery was insane. Absolutely insane. I need to say that. There is an intelligent, independent, adult woman inside of me who cannot believe I'm actually considering doing this."

Jayne was, in her own words, "a Bea Arthur type." She was in her late sixties when she first came to my office. She was the type of person who didn't suffer fools gladly, a tough cookie who came to therapy to engage in some deep but goal-directed introspection. She wanted to feel confident she wasn't making a big mistake by undergoing a cosmetic procedure.

You'll hear about Jayne and her procedure journey later in the book. She's one of a number of former psychotherapy clients you'll meet. Let me be clear about something: none of the clients I have seen in the last twenty-five or so years would recognize their stories in this book. I have very carefully and intentionally altered dates, facts, genders, ages, and all sorts of details in order to protect their privacy. But you will read about real issues that real people confront every day. Knowing a little about the clients will help normalize the struggles you may be experiencing. It will also bring their impressive coping skills and courageous healing processes to life. All of this will help you recognize that you really can maintain your sanity through all stages of the decision-making and procedure processes.

This subject is personally important to me. Like any psychologist, I often recognize pieces of myself in my clients. When I was nineteen, a surgeon eliminated a stuffed nose that had been my near-daily nemesis throughout my childhood. That operation also changed the appearance of my nose forever. The thing is, the primary purpose was not cosmetic. This is important. I believe I was only able to accept the aesthetic aspect of it because there was an undeniable medical component. I remember feeling the need to justify the procedure in that way. The choice to have a strictly cosmetic "nose job" would have felt feminine.

I was particularly concerned about femininity. I was a young gay male who did not identify to myself or to others as either gay or feminine. Although I have grown since then, and the world has also grown, all people considering a cosmetic procedure recognize that it is a public decision. People will notice.

My identity as a psychologist also compels me to be mindful of how others see me. From my clothing choices to my hair color to whether I seem to have altered my body somehow, it's important that I consider the messages I send to my clients through my own behaviors. Some of the people I treat are preparing for a cosmetic procedure, so if I look like I have had that experience, I might seem better able to help them. On the other hand, I also treat people who suffer from an unhealthy desire to alter themselves. It might be unhelpful to my work with those people if they perceive me to have an unhealthy preoccupation in this regard. Like a lot of my clients, how I present to others will be viewed through a particular lens because of the work I do. This is why I have a personal interest in these issues. These decisions have very real and meaningful impacts on our lives.

You Are Not Alone

You might be surprised to learn how many people undergo cosmetic procedures. In 2019, more than 18 million cosmetic procedures were performed in the United States, according to the American Society of Plastic Surgeons. That marks a notable increase from the 12.1 million procedures performed in 2008. Noninvasive treatments such as Botox and fillers far outnumber invasive procedures. The most common invasive procedure was nose reshaping, followed by eyelid surgery, breast augmentation, liposuction, and facelift.

People often think the boom has involved mainly actors, models, and their many admirers in places like Los Angeles and New York City. Nope. The fact is, this has occurred all over the country and world. Miami has the most plastic surgeons per capita of any US city. Yet Salt Lake City, Seattle, San Jose, New Orleans, and Denver are all examples of cities where many cosmetic procedures are performed each year. A lot of cosmetic work is also being done throughout Europe and in many other nations such as Colombia, Brazil, South Korea, Thailand, and Japan.

The good news is that these patients tend to feel quite satisfied with the results. The online site Realself.com boasts over 400,000 verified member reviews. Members are individuals who have undergone a cosmetic procedure. They are asked to submit a "Worth It Rating" focused on their experience. According to Worth It data from 2021, the overwhelming majority of patients indicated they would choose to undergo their chosen procedure again. 2021 Worth It ratings of some common procedures include abdominoplasties (tummy tucks)(95%), breast augmentations/reductions (97%), blepharoplasties (eye lid surgeries)(94%), liposculpture (liposuction)(94%), and rhinoplasties (nose surgeries)(92%) (https://www.realself.com/most-worth-it).

Unsurprisingly, cosmetic work has become big business for physicians. It is marketed throughout the world. Infomercials, docudramas, media coverage, and massive advertising campaigns all enthusiastically offer the promise of improving the bodies we eagerly put on public display in social media posts and in real life.

But Is This Right for YOU?

Just because millions of people are choosing to change themselves in these ways, it doesn't mean it's the right choice for you. I've spent many hours helping clients decide whether to undergo a procedure. That's what led me to write this book. Everyone is unique. The decision whether to go forward with (or forego) a given intervention is a difficult and personal one. We're going to devote a lot of time and effort toward helping you find the path forward that fits best for you.

Right now, you may be at the stage Jayne was when I met her, still only in the considering phase of planning. Or you may have already decided to undergo a cosmetic procedure. This book is intended to help you regardless of which of these groups you're in. There are certain important issues to weigh when contemplating whether to undergo any cosmetic surgical procedure. This book will assist you in evaluating those issues. It will help you feel confident that you've found the right way forward, whatever that way is.

Terminology

Let's talk about terminology for a minute. "Plastic surgery" is a broad term that refers to procedures that alter a person's appearance in some way. Within the realm of plastic surgical procedures, "cosmetic" ones are distinguished from "reconstructive" ones. Cosmetic procedures—such as nose jobs, face-lifts, tummy tucks, liposuction, and facial chemical peels—are elective. People choose these not because their appearance is abnormal or dysfunctional, but rather because it looks different than the way they would prefer to look.

Reconstructive procedures are also cosmetic in the sense that they typically do alter the way a person looks. However, the term "reconstructive" is used because these procedures correct disfigurement due to a variety of factors such as illnesses, birth defects, and accidents. Reconstructive procedures often achieve truly remarkable and life-altering outcomes. Think, for instance, of a person who was born with a prominent facial deformity, or was disfigured by a fire, an animal attack, or a large cancerous tumor.

The purpose of this book is to help both reconstructive and cosmetic procedure patients proceed through the process in a psychologically healthy way. Given the life-altering potential of these procedures, it is particularly important that patients manage their pre- and postprocedure hopes and fears.

To simplify our discussion, I will use the term "cosmetic" broadly and loosely. Since reconstructive procedures often produce visible "cosmetic" changes, I will use the term "cosmetic" to refer to any medical procedure that alters a person's appearance. The content in this book is directed at and will be equally applicable to both reconstructive and purely cosmetic procedure patients.

A Healthy State of Mind

A healthy state of mind helps a patient maintain reasonable expectations for a cosmetic surgical procedure, leaving room for the reality that human bodies are unpredictable, and so also are surgical outcomes. This kind of mindset lays the foundation for a psychologically successful surgical outcome. A perfectionistic and overly demanding mindset is unhealthy and can undermine the work of even the most skillful physicians.

Beau came to me for psychotherapy when he was twenty-five years old. By that time, he had already become a highly sought-after interior designer. Beau had a keen and distinct sense of color and proportion, and his psychotherapy frequently focused on his uncompromising aesthetic and the consequences of his firm views. He often rejected clients, even famous and wealthy ones, because he was unwilling to attach his name to their aesthetic vision.

It fits with his profile that Beau decided he wanted a nose job when he was a teenager, though he didn't get around to undergoing one until much later. "When it comes to proportion, I've always had a strange kind of laser focus," he explained. "A novelist friend says she is unable to read even a Facebook post without fixing word choices in her head. I have a similar problem when I look at certain images. I cannot look at a physical space without seeing deficits and ways to improve it. I have the same problem with outfits people wear. I think I'm most distracted by bad plastic surgery. It's a problem in Los Angeles because so many people have made such outlandish plastic surgery choices. As an interior designer, I see them every day. Many of them are my clients. Their visual ensemble can launch me into a sort of trancelike state. I'm afraid it's noticeable, sometimes."

"So, you feel distracted by it. Can you explain a little more? Maybe give me an example?" I asked.

Beau's response was as prompt as it was precise: "Fillers are the worst. You know, that feline look. They choose it! That distracts me. I find myself commenting in my mind, 'Oh honey, *what* were you thinking?' I can't bring myself to truly believe any person would choose that. It troubles me, actually."

"What troubles you about it?"

"I'm not sure I can say. You know, some people can't resist scratching an itch or clipping a hanging cuticle. That's how I feel when I see something I find visually unappealing. I focus on it to the point of distraction and disturbance."

The issue of distraction arose again when I asked Beau to discuss his feelings about the rhinoplasty he intended to undergo. Beau explained: "I do really dislike looking at my nose. Sometimes, when I see myself in mirrors, I find myself transported as if to another place. All I can do at those times is think ugly thoughts about how my nose looks. I realize this is unhealthy. I literally bully myself in certain moments, relentlessly."

In speaking with Beau about his nose, it was immediately clear he had strong and particular feelings about it. Some therapists might diagnose Beau as compulsive, or with the similar but more severe difficulty known as obsessive-compulsive disorder. Still other therapists might consider his preoccupation with the shape of his nose to be a symptom of the psychological condition known as body dysmorphic disorder. I disagree with all of those views.

If a defined aesthetic sense were a sufficient basis for the diagnosis of a psychological disorder, many of the most brilliant artists in the world could be diagnosed with one. Beau didn't have a disorder. He was gifted with an extraordinarily complex, if uncompromising, visual and spatial processing ability, and that ability influenced how he saw the world. It's not surprising that it also happened to influence his view of the nose on his face.

His impressive visual and spatial processing ability notwithstanding, Beau did have a compulsive tendency that needed curbing. His compulsiveness revealed itself when he searched for a surgeon. Beau interviewed several well-qualified surgeons before choosing one. He was meticulous in his process of assessing whether the surgeon would meet his needs. He carefully examined each surgeon's before-and-after photos and also how each surgeon responded to his questions.

When Beau finally made his choice, he reported he felt completely affirmed during the consultation. The surgeon he chose immediately recognized the ways in which Beau believed his nose to be aesthetically flawed. To Beau's delight, the surgeon affirmed that Beau's observations were accurate and explained precisely how the cosmetic issues could be addressed in a fairly uncomplicated surgical procedure.

Beau's surgical procedure and recovery both went smoothly. His surgeon was pleased with the outcome. Of course, the surgeon's opinion isn't the most important one to me. The real test would be what Beau thought. This would be a test of my belief that Beau's persnickety aesthetic sense was not symptomatic of a severe psychological disorder.

I was happy to learn from Beau that he shared his surgeon's satisfaction with the outcome. I always encourage clients to devote some sessions after the procedure to exploring how they are experiencing the cosmetic changes. Beau chose to do that.

"Now that I like my nose," he explained, "I notice my thoughts have changed. The inner bully is pretty much silent. In fairness, some of that is the result of our work together. I recognize now that the harshness of my inner voice was unhealthy."

"I'm really glad to know you're changing that. So, it sounds like the precision of your aesthetic hasn't changed, but the harsh judgment you often attached to it is softening. Is that an accurate description?"

"Yes. Exactly. In general, it's been helpful to walk around with an awareness of the value of mindfulness. It's helped me to remain more aware of my intention to lead with kindness in my relations with other people. Using a brief mindfulness and breathing exercise repeatedly throughout the day has been very helpful in that way."

"I'm so happy to hear about these steps forward," I said. "After a procedure like the one you had, I always also like to ask the client about their experience of looking into mirrors. Has that experience changed in any ways?"

"It's funny you ask about that," Beau replied. "I do notice a change. I guess the best way to explain it is I notice that I actually look at myself in the mirror, now. Prior to the procedure, I had grown accustomed to *glancing* at mirrors but not looking carefully into them, if that makes sense. You remember I told you how distracted I would get when I would look at my nose? I used to avoid looking carefully at my face, because of my nose. I could see details like whether the buttons on my shirt were fastened correctly, without ever looking at my nose. I'm not glancing at mirrors anymore. I'm looking directly into them. I'm not making an effort to avoid seeing my nose. As melodramatic as it may sound, it feels freeing and very empowering."

"I don't think it sounds melodramatic. It's actually pretty common for people to feel persecuted by mirrors. You may have seen the framed quote I have in my office that says, 'Better to allow mirrors to suffer from disuse than misuse.' I discuss that idea a lot with clients."

Throughout our work together, Beau and I focused on helping him maintain his high standards but not use them to mistreat himself. We discussed his tendency to be so demanding of himself and others. By exploring the way he felt about his nose, we were able to delve deeper into his lifelong tendency to become preoccupied by his reactions and demands.

Over the years, distraction has become a common focus of my work with clients. Distractions sometimes prevent us from being fully present in the moment, with others or with ourselves. This was one of the unhealthy aspects of the distractions impacting Beau. His penchant for sinking deep into intense criticisms continually transported him away from the present moment. His distracted state when he would look at his nose, or at aesthetically displeasing things outside of himself, were examples of this.

Prior to our work together, Beau had not examined his tendency to detach from himself when he would become consumed by criticisms. Likewise, although he knew he was self-critical in some ways, he had not recognized that there is a self-rejection that motivates the detachment from the self. Mindfulness and meditation can be especially beneficial for clients who need to learn to treat themselves better and to remain present with themselves more often. I hope you are beginning to get a sense of why the concept of presence is fundamental to emotional wellness. We will examine this concept in greater detail later in this book.

The desire to change and improve is a natural instinct. It touches all of us at one time or another. The important thing to recognize about Beau is that, although he was self-critical, he was also emotionally well-balanced. His work in psychotherapy helped him learn to take better care of himself and others, but he came to me with a fairly healthy self-image. This enabled him to have reasonable and limited goals for the procedure; his expectations were realistic. When patients have healthy expectations, cosmetic work is much more likely to be successful.

Psychological Health Matters

Hundreds of interesting scientific papers focus on psychological concepts such as happiness, sadness, resilience, life satisfaction, fear, and anxiety.

Although some of these papers are available to the public, most psychological theories never reach the typical non-researcher. What a shame. There is so much we know about how to be happy and why we become sad—some of which I'd like to share in this book as you plan for, undergo, and recover from a surgical procedure.

Effective psychotherapy can be especially important as a person prepares for something as sensitive and potentially life-changing as a permanent alteration of the way they look. One of the ways goal-directed psychotherapy can help is by providing what some people have labeled "life hacks": new ways of coping with life's struggles. They can be applied to various situations. Some examples follow, and others will emerge in later parts of the book.

Healthier Thoughts, Feelings, and Behaviors

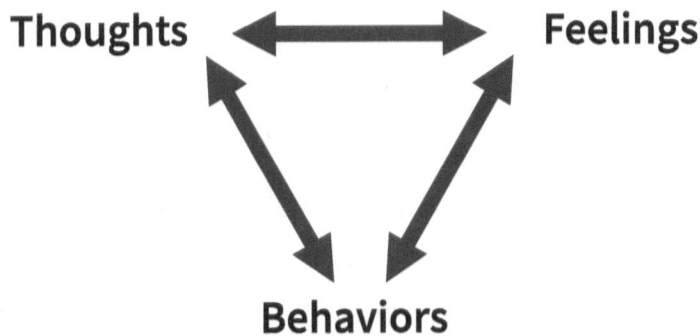

In cognitive behavioral therapy (CBT), one of the fundamental concepts is the idea that the ways we think, feel, and behave are constantly bringing one another into existence. As a simple example, if a person thinks he is ugly, he is more likely to feel feelings such as shame and maybe sadness. And if he thinks and feels those things, he is likely to behave by avoiding people or covering himself.

The core of CBT is the belief that healthier thoughts, feelings, and behaviors help us function better. "Healthy" does not mean positive; it means accurate. CBT combines two types of psychotherapy—cognitive and behavioral. Cognitive therapy focuses on the idea that we cope best with our world when we *think* about it accurately. So, for instance, a surgical outcome the patient didn't want is unfortunate, but if the patient views it accurately, they will not consider it to be catastrophic or intolerable.

Behavioral therapy focuses on the power of healthy *behaviors* to assist a person to live a life with more satisfaction and purpose. It centers on what a person does that impacts how that person feels and thinks. When we work on behavioral aspects of CBT, we focus on the idea that it helps a client do things like eat in healthy ways, exercise, socialize, get enough sleep, engage in leisure activities, and avoid unhealthy behaviors like substance abuse. So, in CBT, the therapist helps the client do both at the same time—adopt healthy thoughts and behaviors.

Cognitive Work

In CBT we often utilize metaphors to help clients *think* differently. For example, a client might compare herself to a ship, and life's stressors to the sea, which is rough sometimes yet calm at other times. On days when the sea is rough and the currents strong, she may struggle to "navigate" safely. She would need to persevere through storms and trust that her vessel will not fall apart.

We can think of rough seas as a metaphor for any of the sources of stress we continually confront in life. We all have to cope with such things as other people's bad behavior, the experience of unfairness and injustice, governmental systems failing us, and the machines in our lives malfunctioning. On the more severe end of the stress continuum, we must cope sometimes with death, illness, disability, and other painful losses.

Maintaining psychological wellness in the face of life's stressors requires good psychological health. This is how the ship metaphor can be useful. It provides a great way to look at ourselves and assess our coping skills. We can think of ourselves as both the ship and as its captain. The person who copes well with harsh weather conditions is someone who accepts them as inevitable, temporary, and largely uncontrollable. In this way, the metaphor reminds us of a fundamental truth: good mental health requires that we accept what *is*.

It's easy—and common—for people to assert that they accept their reality. But people often accept things intellectually while resisting acceptance at a deeper, more authentic level within themselves. We often deceive ourselves to avoid dealing directly with our own pieces of internal resistance. Cognitive-behavioral techniques can help us deal more directly with all aspects of our reality, and this can help us respond to stress in healthier ways.

Behavioral Coping Techniques

Surgical procedures are traumatic to the body. Robust recoveries from surgery are more likely to occur when patients have healthy minds and bodies. This is why healthy behaviors are so important. This book will focus on a variety of behaviors that nurture psychological growth and change. Behavioral exercises alter our behaviors, which tend to bring about changes in our thoughts and feelings. Many people are surprised to learn that meditation is one of the most powerful behavioral exercises, impacting both the way we feel and the way we think. We will explore the power of meditation throughout this book.

Behavioral exercises embrace the notion that in order to cope more effectively, a person must act differently in addition to thinking differently. *We change by changing.* There are many different types of behavioral exercises, but all of them share one thing in common: they require action.

Cognitive and behavioral exercises not only engage us in action but also engage the observer within us. Self-monitoring is a vitally important behavior in maintaining psychological wellness. I have provided a number of exercises that will help you do this, and do it in ways that help preserve your emotional wellness within the context of cosmetic changes.

Meditation: It's Not Just for Relaxing

Meditation is often considered a harmless method of achieving relaxation. I don't think of meditation in that way. I believe meditation and mindfulness are very powerful tools that directly address some deep-seated psychological struggles. When used correctly, meditation and mindfulness can provide not only a sense of calm and self-compassion but also deep insight into the workings of the mind. In this book you will be shown a number of examples of meditations and mindfulness practices that you can use to pursue various goals.

In Chapter 12, I provide a series of twenty-eight meditations, mantras, and affirmations for use in the days prior to and after a cosmetic procedure. These tools can be used to develop a more nurturing mindset. If your planned cosmetic work is already scheduled, you might want to skip forward to Chapter 12 now, so that you can begin using the tools in that chapter even as you read the rest of the book.

Mantras and affirmations empower us through the action of positive self-talk. Healthy guided meditations empower us in similar ways. All three devices—meditation, mantras, and affirmations—expose our brain to positive and empowering ideas. If we are willing to use these tools regularly, and with the intention to integrate the messages into our day-to-day mindset, they will assist us in adopting new ways of thinking and being.

I can illustrate the power of meditations with a personal story. Prior to becoming a psychologist, I was a licensed attorney. When I was studying for the California Bar Exam, I meditated every day. I had read that a thirty-minute daily meditation could refresh the mind and provide an additional three hours of productive study time. I needed all the productive study time I could find. So, during my months of exam preparation, whenever I felt tired while studying, I would pop the guided meditation into my recorder, lie down, and rest while listening to it. The meditation instructed me to picture myself during all phases of taking the exam. It also instructed me to see myself leaving the exam site. I was told to imagine myself feeling overjoyed and confident, certain that I had done well on that particular day.

Sure enough, after day one, I left the exam site overjoyed and full of confidence, certain everything had gone well. I felt jubilant.

There was only one problem: I was fully aware I had not performed well. Fully aware. There was a spring in my step, a smile on my face, and a sensation of joy and satisfaction occupying every cell of my body. Yet I was certain I had not done well. I knew I had not provided a passing response in the essay portion on that first day of the exam. I knew it because I had gambled by not studying a particular legal issue (nuisance law, I think it was, but don't quote me on that; it was a long time ago). That unusual legal issue was rarely tested on the Bar Exam, so I neglected it in favor of preparing for other subjects that were likelier to be on the test. Well, as fate would have it, the Bar examiners devoted an entire question, plus part of another question, to that single legal issue.

As I walked home from the exam site, I knew I had blown it. I knew that completely failing on one of the six major essays, and missing key points on another, would be enough to make me fail the exam. I was certain I was not going to pass.

A few months later, when the results were released, I received the confirmation I expected: I did not pass the Bar Exam. It was administered over three days. As I had suspected, my performance on day one reflected exactly the deficits I suspected it would, and had I performed on that first day as I had on days two and three, I would surely have passed.

In the months that followed, I had no doubt about what went wrong during the exam. I knew what I needed to do to pass the next time. I still, however, felt unsettled and deeply confused by one thing. My mind would repeatedly wander to a nagging mystery: what had gone wrong with my brain *after* the first test day? The jubilation I felt as I left the exam site—what was that about? I have always tended to be drawn to logical and rational thoughts. It troubled me that there was absolutely no logical reason for me to have felt so positive after that first day—I knew it even in the moment. So why did I feel that way?

I continued preparing for the next Bar Exam, still using the meditations often, because I did feel like they bought me a solid couple of hours more of alert study time. One day, after finishing a meditation, a thought occurred to me: "Wait a minute. Could that elation and confidence I felt have been caused by that goofy meditation?" (Sorry for the negativity, but that was how I thought about meditation back then.) I listened to the meditation again and again. I do now believe that's the explanation for my confidence after the exam. And this remains one of the reasons I don't think of meditation as goofy or ridiculous anymore.

The thing that still blows me away about meditation is the way it works. It didn't brainwash me. I wasn't delusional as I left the exam. If I had been delusional, I might have believed I did fabulously. But I didn't believe that; instead, I just felt good, even though the exam had not gone well. So the meditation's impact was powerful, yet it did not alter my reality. It altered my perception of my reality—my interpretation of it. I believed I'd have to take the exam again, but I trusted I was going to be okay in spite of that.

Meditation, when practiced regularly, can produce positive changes like this. Changes that sort of sneak up on you. The meditations in this book serve various functions, but all of them will help you prepare your body and mind for a successful cosmetic outcome and more self-compassion in general.

Using Journals in Healthy Ways

Journaling is a type of behavioral exercise that helps us look more carefully at ourselves. You will encounter journaling exercises in several places in this book. The first exercise is at the end of this chapter. Journals provide the writer a chance to explore and clarify thoughts and feelings. When used wisely, journals also offer the writer an empowering source of support and validation. Journals help a person feel heard and affirmed, the way we do when a close friend supportively listens to us. This process is often cathartic, enabling us to transform and resolve thoughts and feelings in ways that mere thinking typically doesn't.

As you engage in journaling, it's good to remember something: a journal is a tool. Any tool can be harmful if used incorrectly. With this in mind, here are some suggestions for using a journal therapeutically:

1. Choose a journal you will look forward to opening at the end of the day.

2. Fill your journal with positive but accurate sentiments. Imagine you are writing to a friend, telling them whatever you need to say.

3. Be *honest*. Try not to worry about offending someone. This journal is *yours*. *You* are its only reader.

4. Be accurate. Don't minimize your feelings, but don't exaggerate them either.

5. If you notice an irresistible pull to write only about critical and unhopeful thoughts and feelings, *do it*. Get them out of your system. Then do the following:

   a. Think of these sections as "garbage dumps." You could even label them that way in the margin. Use them like waste containers into which you dump ugly, nonconstructive thoughts.

   b. Imagine yourself physically removing this negativity from your mind.

   c. When you notice yourself writing about qualities, traits, emotions, or characteristics that carry negative connotations—fear, distrust, cynicism, anger, critical thoughts—try to follow them up with alternative, countervailing ideas. This is not about lying. It's about maintaining balance and accuracy. For example:

      I dread seeing Rose after I have my neck wrinkles eliminated. I know she will notice and comment. And it will be in a disparaging way. She always makes me feel like a fool.

This could be followed up by writing something like:

   Rose will always have a corrective comment —about everything. I have to remember that I don't need Rose's approval. I know so many people who will be supportive. I need to stop giving Rose so much power.

Brief Screening Tools

You will find simple, short screening tools throughout this book. These can be used to help you identify opportunities for growth. After choosing your responses and scoring your results, it's best to then go back and look at each of your answers. Try to be curious about what they tell you about yourself. It also can be helpful to bring your responses to a meeting with a mental health professional who can assist you in exploring the information that lies within them.

 Journaling Exercise: Hope and Change

To explore what you would be seeking in a cosmetic procedure, try journaling about the broad questions below. Try to allow yourself to set your own rules regarding how you respond. Do what feels helpful to you. For instance, if you find yourself feeling overwhelmed by the breadth and depth of your responses, try cutting back on the level of detail or the time you devote to each response. You can continue to process your responses by returning to them at another time and, after re-reading them, continuing to process them while writing more or while walking or engaging in some other form of movement. You could also continue to process your journal entries by bringing them with you to a therapy appointment and using them as a starting point in a dialogue with your therapist (this is a great idea for any of the journaling exercises in this book).

It's also important to note that journaling can be emotionally exhausting. A journaling exercise sometimes leads to feelings that are so intense they interrupt the writing, If this happens and you feel unable to focus on the intended subject of the entry, you can shift the focus of your writing to the feelings themselves. Describe the emotions that are being activated and then discuss the content in a session with a mental health professional.

If I have the procedure and it goes well, what change(s) in myself do I seek?

1. Physical (how I appear):

2. Emotional (how I feel):

3. Cognitive (how I think):

4. Behavioral (how I behave):

Meditations

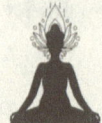

Exercise: Breath-Focused Mindfulness Meditation

There are several methods you can use for this and other guided meditations in this book. First, you could use my voice to guide you via the recordings I have online. Another option would be to keep the written instructions in front of you and follow one instruction at a time, returning to the book once you have completed each instruction. Or, you could record yourself reading the instructions and then use your own recorded voice to guide you through the meditation. If you do this, be sure to leave plenty of time between each instruction.

There are many forms of meditation. The following is a breath-focused form of mindfulness meditation. As you do it, please consider the following practice tips:

1. The objective is presence and awareness, not peacefulness. Try to coexist with your breath and with all your feelings and perceptions, even the rejecting, intolerant ones.

2. When meditating, expect your attention to wax and wane. This is normal. Try to be aware. When you notice your mind roaming, such as by judging, pondering, problem-solving, or engaging in other forms of thinking, try to gently remind yourself of the objective and refocus on your breath as best you can.

3. The length of the meditation is up to you. Even one minute is a good start.

4. Remember that this is a practice of simply *being*, rather than *doing*.

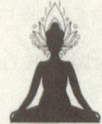

Instructions for the Breath-Focused Mindfulness Meditation:

> **Note:** You may follow the instructions, below, or access a guided version of this meditation at DrAlanGoodwin.com.

1. Find a quiet, private place. This will be a brief version of this meditation to demonstrate the technique but you can make this meditation much longer, if you'd like. And I encourage you to do that, when you feel ready.

2. Assume a comfortable, relaxed, alert position; upright, but not stiff. If you prefer lying down, that's o.k. but try to also practice this meditation sitting up sometimes so that you can compare the experiences and choose whichever is most helpful to you. Remember, the goal is awareness and presence.

3. Begin by breathing in a relaxed, normal way.

4. Close your eyes or leave your them open but resting on a single object rather than your eyes being in active use.

5. Notice whatever your five senses reveal to you. Take your time.

6. Just breathe. Slowly in and slowly out. Devote this time to stopping and just being present with your breath. Simply take slow, deep breaths in and out.

7. You may choose to pause a beat after you inhale and then enjoy a nice long exhale. Normally, it is relaxing to exhale a bit longer than you inhale.

8. Remain focused on your breathing. Simply notice each time you inhale and each time you exhale.

9. To help you focus on your breathing, attach the number "one" to each breath in and attach the number "two" to each breath out. In your mind hear those numbers as you breathe. If you prefer, say the numbers aloud and quietly to yourself while you breathe. One. Two. One. Two.

10. If your mind wanders and engages thoughts, notice that, accept that it happened, and then gently remind yourself to focus only on your breath.

11. Try to allow breathing to be enough. Allow thoughts to float into and then out of your mind. Try not to focus on the content of those thoughts. You can do that later. For now, just focus on your breaths.

12. When you feel ready to end the meditation, devote a few breaths to gratitude. Inhale feelings of gratitude. As you exhale, say a mantra or two silently or quietly, such as: *I am learning*, or *I am growing*, or *I feel blessed.*

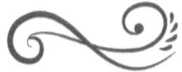

CHAPTER 2

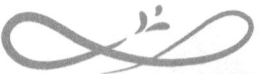

What Does the Buddha Have to Do with YOUR Surgery?

The mind is everything. What you think, you become.

— Buddha

Meltdown

"I had a meltdown, doc. A total meltdown. I'm lucky I'm even here tonight. Sorry to jump right in this way, but I need to examine this." George was a decent, friendly, considerate, and normally well-mannered thirty-nine-year-old man. He was an introvert with an engineering background, working as an architect. He sought psychotherapy to address symptoms of depression and anxiety. Like a lot of people who struggle with those symptoms, George also struggled with anger management. He tended to be pretty hard on people, especially himself. He also happened to be preparing to undergo a liposuction procedure.

George continued, "So, I'm driving on Pico, near the 405. It's the middle of the afternoon but, of course, Pico was congested for no reason. It was hotter than hell outside and I was late for a meeting, a meeting I didn't even want to attend." George paused to take a swig of water from his teal, Kirkland thermos. He stopped and leaned back on the couch. He took a breath in and then a long exhale. I had suggested he use this breathing technique to help him maintain calmness and self-control in difficult moments. It's a great way to reset yourself, like restarting your computer when it seems to be overwhelmed.

When George continued, he labored to resist raising his voice. It was clear he was trying to manage his activation level. "So, I'm in the left turn lane, okay? And there's a guy in front of me. He's first in line and I'm second. This is the *left* turn lane. So, the light turns green, but he doesn't move. He waits, and waits, and waits. No moving, okay? Until the light turns yellow and then the light turns red. And then you know what he did? The same thing. He didn't move. He just sat there. Now, you have to remember, I'm already running late."

"I understand. Sounds frustrating," I said. "So, even though he was in the turn lane and traffic had cleared, he didn't turn."

George leaned forward on the couch. His energy was intensifying, despite the breath work. "Right! He stayed *in* the lane even *after* the light had been green for an entire cycle. Exactly! Now, I'll give the guy this: traffic wasn't clear. The oncoming traffic was stopped the whole time. They were all bumper-to-bumper. But listen—and this is important—the guy never inched. He never INCHED!"

"I'm sorry, George," I interjected. "Inched? I'm not sure what you mean."

"In that situation," George explained, "you *inch*! You INCH! You inch your car forward and turn the wheel a little toward the left. You do that as a signal. And then someone in the traffic facing you moves a little forward and someone else moves a little backward. They make room for you to get through. You *ask* people to create a little *space*. He could have inched and found room to squeeze through. If *he* had done *that*, then *I* could have followed. But he didn't. So, I couldn't."

"Okay. I understand what you mean now," I said.

"But we're just getting started. Are you ready? He did that for three full light sequences. He didn't inch at all for *three* lights. Three!"

"Wow. Three lights?"

"THREE LIGHTS," George confirmed. "Now, I admit it, when the third red light came, I lost it. I just lost it. I don't know what came over me. I literally got out of my car and raced up to his window. I stood at his window and knocked on it and yelled at him like a maniac. I think I was saying things like, 'What are you doing?' and 'You're a terrible driver!' and 'You need to create space!' To be honest, I'm not even sure what I said. I was like stuck in a thick fog of rage. I was literally out of my mind for about thirty seconds."

"Yikes," I said. "So, what happened next?"

"Well, luckily, I was the only lunatic. He was a terrible driver, but apparently he wasn't a lunatic. So, I stood there, waving my arms and yelling, and he just looked at me through his closed window and started cracking up. I don't blame him. I was literally out of my mind and body. Something about his laughing jolted me back to reality. I suddenly realized I was standing in the middle of Pico, wondering how I'd gotten there and where to go next. I decided it was time to return to my powder-blue Prius and contemplate the ass I'd made of myself." George exhaled and relaxed back into the armchair, shaking his head. "So, eventually the light turned green, traffic cleared, he turned, I turned, and nothing else happened. I was late for my meeting but, surprisingly, the sky didn't fall in."

"That's pretty intense, George."

"You're not kidding," George muttered.

"It's good that you brought it in to talk about. It's courageous of you to share all those details."

"I'll tell you the craziest part," George said, leaning up. "Do you know what I would have done if he had gotten out of his car? If you do know, maybe you can tell *me*, because I have no idea. I wasn't gonna fight with the guy. I haven't actually physically fought with someone since I was about six. Anyway, fighting with strangers isn't my M.O. No, I fight with *myself*. I keep my rage on the inside, where it can punish me and, over time, cause my organs to prematurely decompose. I play the long game, that way." Again, George paused. The sarcasm and intensity seemed to drain out of him as he slumped back into the armchair. When he continued, his voice was quiet and he sounded sad and dejected. "Anyway, if that guy had gotten out of his car, I might have gotten myself killed. It scares the hell out of me that I was so out of my mind."

As I mentioned, George was like a lot of people in that his depressive symptoms often got expressed in anger and irritability. As the old adage says, "It feels better to be mad than sad." We all want to feel safe. People, and especially men, often associate sadness with weakness, and anger with strength and safety. In this way, anger is often used as a defense against feelings of vulnerability.

The Tool of Mindfulness

Anger is a reactive emotion, one reaction among many other choices. Mindfulness is a tool we can use to examine the choices we make to think and feel and behave in certain ways. George's decision to exhibit anger is an example of this.

It may sound strange to describe someone *deciding* to exhibit anger. For many people, anger is more of a reflex than a choice. But we can acquire more control over our anger and other emotions. Mindfulness and meditation are tools for achieving that.

As a male psychologist offering solution-focused psychotherapy, I've seen a lot of clients like George. It's not uncommon for people with anger issues to seek out a male therapist. The experiences with my clients suggest this is because they assume a man will be less likely to harshly judge their anger. I'm not sure that's true, but regardless, they come to me knowing they have a behavior problem they need to fix.

I've seen many clients with anger issues profoundly benefit from solution-focused psychotherapy integrated with mindfulness and meditation practices. This is why I present meditations throughout this book and why, in Chapter 12, I offer a series of daily meditations that are specifically designed to assist cosmetic surgery patients.

Believe it or not, George's anger is particularly relevant in a book about coping with cosmetic medical procedures. Patients who tend to be overly reactive have more difficulty with the unpredictability of cosmetic outcomes. Effective psychotherapy can tame the reactivity. I have found Eastern ideas and the practice of meditation to be potent tools in psychotherapy.

In this chapter, you will notice my giving credit to Buddhist teachers. I want to acknowledge that these concepts have been articulated in myriad forms and in many different religious traditions and cultures. I credit the sources I relied upon. The concepts are broad and can supplement any spiritual tradition, including the absence of one.

What Is Mindfulness?

Mindfulness enhances so many activities. Yoga instructors encourage their students to be mindful as they engage in their yoga practice. Corporate consultants cite mindfulness as contributing to positive outcomes in workforce morale, motivation, performance levels, and creativity. All of these directly influence and benefit the bottom line (profits), which explains the growing presence of mindfulness practices in workplaces.

The concept of mindfulness has existed for thousands of years. Recently, mindfulness beliefs and practices have exploded in popularity in the West. Contemporary Buddhists such as Pema Chödrön and Thich Nhat Hanh, plus several non-Buddhists, have helped many Westerners recognize the central role these practices can play in helping a person live a healthy and happy life.

When I refer to mindfulness, I am referring simply to the conscious awareness of one's experience of any situation. This refers to how a person is feeling, thinking, and behaving in that moment. Mindfulness is about seeing our experience, in the moment, exactly as it is. Sometimes, mindfulness is defined as a nonjudgmental observation. I don't define it that way. We judge sometimes. As an emotional wellness tool, one of the most powerful aspects of mindfulness is that it encourages us to make room for all parts of ourselves, even the judgmental parts.

The Unnatural Practice of Meditation

Mindfulness meditation sounds like such an easy practice. It requires simply focusing on your breath while remaining aware of your sensations and perceptions. The goal is to remain present with your immediate experiences.

People often describe meditation as a tool for relaxing. Although relaxation is sometimes a pleasant byproduct of mindfulness meditation, relaxation isn't the goal. Awareness, or *presence*, is the goal. Presence isn't always relaxing. In fact, it's often pretty stressful to feel present, particularly when being present involves preparing for a surgical procedure.

The discomfort of being present is a common reason why people feel frustration and anxiety when they try to meditate. I've had several clients who made a plan to begin a regular meditation practice only to abandon it soon after starting. George was one of those people.

When I discussed George's experience of trying to meditate, he said, "I just can't do it. It's my fault. My mind is just too active to allow me to meditate. I start to think about a work project, and then a conversation I had with someone, and then the lawnmower outside, and it never ends. So it just stresses me out. I feel like a failure. My mind is always way too full of thoughts." And so, initially, George gave up, thinking he just didn't have the right constitution to meditate correctly.

Some clients refuse to try again. George didn't refuse. He tried again and again and he eventually succeeded. Ultimately, he realized that we *all* have very busy minds. He needed to embrace this aspect of his humanity. In time, George learned to stop trying to silence his mind and instead used meditation to practice noticing and peacefully coexisting with his hectic and random thoughts.

Meditation and Our Reactive Mind

If you doubt we are genetically inclined to have active minds, think for a minute about our shared history. I'm talking about our distant history here. I'm not an anthropologist, but my understanding is *Homo sapiens* began walking the earth around 300,000 years ago. Those ancestors confronted any number of threats to their safety. The people who survived were the ones who were alert and reactive to threats. That ability to perceive threats and then respond appropriately required an active mind, which we inherited.

It follows that a mind that is active, in the sense of being responsive to perceived threats, is a distractible mind. So, our inherited active brain makes us susceptible to distraction, including by our own thoughts. Originally, the distractibility was a survival skill. Today we are preoccupied by distractions too much of the time. This is especially true of people who struggle with anxiety.

One of the objectives in meditation is to train your brain to be less distractible. For a lot of reasons, that's not easy to do. Think of our ancestors again. We feel alert and aware when we are distractible, and this causes us to feel safer. We like to feel safe, so we like being distractible.

But distractibility is sort of like caffeine. A little of it is energizing, but too much of it is anxiety-provoking and addictive. Like caffeine, it's uncomfortable to try to reduce distractibility, especially if you've relied on a lot of it.

All of this explains why meditation tends to be unpleasant, at least at first. Meditation challenges us to interrupt our habitual tendency toward distraction. This doesn't feel natural or comfortable to most people.

Meditation gives us practice taming our overly active minds. There is a very good reason why we would want to do this: our present world, most of the time, doesn't require immediate reactivity in order to preserve our safety. Sure, like our ancestors, we do need to make quick decisions, a lot of them, but not as many or as quickly as that anxious part of our brain thinks we do. We meditate because our habitual level of reactivity is unhealthy. It fuels anxiety disorders, depression, and other problems.

The goal of meditation is to get healthier by being more present. When we learn how to resist the excessive reactivity, we acquire more time with ourselves. During those extra moments, we can more mindfully choose our reactions. In this way, mindfulness meditation helps us learn to value *being*, rather than just *doing*.

Meditation and its Relevance to Cosmetic Surgery

The practice of meditation has a particular application to cosmetic procedures. Cosmetic patients sometimes feel overwhelmed by strong feelings and thoughts. Much like George after the traffic light had turned red for the third time, cosmetic patients sometimes feel compelling urges to take action in response to their impulses. The problem is the impulsive actions are often ill-advised. For instance, a patient may ignore their surgeon's healing instructions, thereby increasing the risk of a poor outcome.

A meditation practice can help a patient prepare for the procedure and the recovery period. This can reduce impulsiveness and other forms of self-sabotage. With practice, meditation creates more *space* in a patient's mind. In psychological terms, this can be thought of as simply adding more time between stimuli and our responses to them. The space created by meditation can help us to respond more mindfully, guided less by fear and more by self-compassion.

George's Tiny "Space"

The space between experiencing a thought and then responding to that thought became a very helpful concept for George. A mindfulness meditation practice enabled him to gradually buy himself more time before reacting to his thoughts and emotions. For example, think about his experience in that left turn lane. A space of even an extra second or two provides someone like George the opportunity to stop, breathe, and choose a response that is not dominated by a sense of urgency and the perception that someone has disrespected him. In other words, it allows for a less personalized way of experiencing things and responding to them.

This also played a role during George's liposuction experience. Like many people who struggle with depression, George was sometimes deeply unkind toward himself. He tended to be harshly critical of his weight, his body, his personality, and anything else he associated with himself. A number of times leading up to the day of the procedure, George and I shared exchanges like this one:

"I'm canceling it."

"Why don't we talk about what's going on, George?"

"I feel ridiculous. I'm five foot five and I weigh 230 pounds. This procedure is not going to change that. Not much, anyway. I feel like a fool."

"Help me understand," I said. "When you decided on this procedure, you felt those feelings, but you said you expected the procedure to help kick-start an exercise program. You said you knew patients who had succeeded in doing that."

"Yeah, I know. It's a waste of time. I don't know what I was thinking." George sat back and paused, looking out the window. His body seemed to release some of the intensity, and he became more pensive, his voice quieter. He continued, "I went to the gym today. I look ridiculous. I will never belong there."

"Did something happen today to cause you to feel that way? Or was it just unpleasant in general?"

"Both. I always have both. First of all, I always feel invisible there. No, that's wrong. I don't feel invisible. I feel the opposite. I feel completely visible but entirely irrelevant and like I don't belong there. And there is not a person in the gym who doesn't see me that way. I stick out like a sore thumb. I need to quit going to gyms. You know, I see people there talking and socializing. Do you know how many times someone has ever said a word to me? Never. Never once. Women literally walk around weight racks to avoid me."

George had a tendency to sink into these ways of thinking and feeling. Depression is sadness, and it does this to people. The focus is often on loss and deficit. A sense of personal inadequacy is also common in people who feel depressed. George tended to believe other people were a lot more skilled and fortunate than he was. In some ways, of course, he was right. But we can all say that. We all have our limitations and the personal struggles that emerge from them. Effective treatment for depression isn't about taking away the struggles; it's about helping the person lessen the discomfort of them. A person like George needs to see the world just differently enough to recognize opportunities to find happiness.

Much of the work in our solution-focused psychotherapy was aimed at showing George how abusively he tended to treat himself. The overly critical ways of thinking about himself and about other people were toxic and inaccurate. So, some of the work was about helping him see that there are healthier, more balanced ways of thinking.

Identifying new ways of thinking is the cognitive part of the work. It tends to be pretty straightforward; it simply focuses on being accurate. Things get more complicated when the psychotherapy process turns toward implementing new ways of thinking. Meditation provides an opportunity to practice noticing long-held, habitual ways of thinking. Noticing the thoughts begins the process of changing them.

Over time, meditation helped George practice slowing down his reactions to the world. This created "space" for alternative interpretations of events. For instance, George might consider alternative ways of thinking about the other people at the gym. Maybe they didn't dislike him or reject him; maybe they were just shy or lacking in confidence, unable to try to make a new friend by approaching George. Or maybe they thought George's shyness meant he wanted to be left alone. But George's mind had too little "space" to allow room for these or other alternative interpretations.

Another piece of the work I did with George is particularly relevant to cosmetic procedures. In the process of trying to help George open his mind to other ways of thinking, during the same session discussed earlier, I said, "So, George, the gym experience today is leading you to consider not only quitting the gym but also canceling the liposuction operation?"

"Yes. It is. It's a waste of time and money. Besides, I keep having crazy thoughts. This will sound ridiculous, but I keep thinking about the doctor and nurses seeing my body, and it's really bothering me. It first occurred to me the other night. They'll all be looking at me. I just never really thought about that. Even when I took pictures at the surgeon's office, I sort of held my stomach in a little. It's all just really embarrassing. I know I'll be anesthetized and I'll never know what they say or think, but it bothers me. I know that sounds crazy, but it does bother me."

"I don't think it sounds crazy," I said. "I think it's understandable that you would think that way. I think your expectation about how they will think about you and your body is a projection. I think you're expecting them to think about you in the same harsh and critical ways that you do."

George replied, "I don't doubt that, but I'm being honest."

"I think you're being honest, too, and it's really helpful to our work. Because it's toxic and abusive, George. The disrespect you feel toward your body is something we really need to continue to explore, whether you undergo the procedure or not."

These instances with George are typical of the way mindfulness can help a person hear what they tend to say to themselves. A person's inner dialogue has a powerful impact on their state of mind and this directly influences their feelings and their behaviors. Before a person can change their thoughts, they need to hear them, evaluate them, and then identify what needs to change.

Mindfulness Meditation for Nurturing Self-Compassion

Someone like George has been practicing being unkind toward himself for decades. Changing those patterns takes time and the right kind of work. A regular meditation practice, combined with cognitive work, helped him begin to hear his inner dialogue differently.

Like most people, George found this difficult to do. He didn't want to coexist with his body as it was. For a while, he resisted the fundamental idea that, in order to change his body, he was going to have to accept and embrace it.

This is why mindfulness meditation is so powerful for someone like George. All people who struggle with depression struggle with intolerance. There are things about their life that they reject. Meditation gives us practice coexisting with those things instead of rejecting them. Coexisting doesn't take away the struggle, but if done right, it does take away the suffering.

Of course, it's hard to coexist with people and things that we wish would disappear. And this is why effective mindfulness meditation encourages self-compassion. Self-compassion occurs when we honor our struggles. By looking at our struggles in this way, such as the struggle with intolerance, we make room for seeing our intolerance with curiosity. Curiosity is the key to transforming intolerance into acceptance.

Initially, George agreed to use writing exercises to examine his anger toward his body. Like most of us, his rejection of his body was influenced by the images and messages we all see so frequently. He also spoke about body-shaming experiences he'd had as a child.

The cognitive part of our work together focused on the ways he had come to think about his size. There was an intolerance he felt toward people he labeled "fat." He labeled himself that way. We carefully explored the origins of his harsh judgments.

Mindfulness meditation urges us to embrace the ethic of nonviolence. This includes violence against all aspects of ourselves—our bodies, our thoughts, our feelings, and any other aspect. George agreed to use meditations to practice sitting with himself. This helped him notice his inclination to reject himself.

The work of loving ourselves as we are unfolds over time. George's success was no different. It occurred progressively. Over a period of months, he began to adopt new ways of thinking and feeling about himself. He reinforced those changes in his meditation practice. As I alluded to earlier, he also used brief breathing exercises to enable himself to stop and alter the condemning and overly reactive ways of being that had become habitual. He actively changed his self-talk as well. By replacing critical inner dialogue with self-affirming mantras, like the ones in the meditations in Chapter 12, George gradually succeeded in changing the way he felt about himself.

At the end of this chapter, you will find a loving kindness meditation that focuses on self-compassion. It can be used at any time of day or night. George used it before bedtime in support of his sleep hygiene routine. Some people report that bedtime meditations like this contribute to more peaceful dreams and a more pleasant waking experience in the morning.

Meditation and the Fish Within You

One issue I'd like to address is your mindset while meditating. We've discussed the common misperception that meditation requires an absence of thoughts. On the contrary, mindfulness meditation presupposes you will have lots of thoughts and gives you practice coexisting with them. Since that's so difficult to do, I want to share a tool for practicing it.

I recommend that when you meditate, you imagine you are a fish. Yep, a fish. Any fish. You can be a flounder, a perch, a walleye, a rainbow trout—whatever you prefer.

As you meditate, envision yourself as the fish, swimming through the water. Imagine that you are surrounded by baited hooks. The baited hooks are metaphorical images of your thoughts. When we meditate, thoughts pop into our minds constantly. We are surrounded by delicious, enticing thoughts, and we feel drawn to them in the same way a fish feels drawn to baited hooks.

For example, as you meditate, you might suddenly think, "I wish I hadn't said what I said to Marco earlier today." If you indulge that thought, you will soon have a related thought, like, "If I had simply said X instead, Marco would never have said Y, and then I would not have said Z, and we would not have gotten into that big argument."

Do you see how, when you indulge or engage a thought, you initiate a series of other thoughts? In this way, engaging a thought is like a fish biting a baited hook. Once you take the bait and engage the thought, you can expect to be controlled by that thought just like a fish is controlled as it's dragged around by a hook in its mouth. Once we take the bait, our thoughts mercilessly yank us from one thought to another.

The good news is there are ways to feel less dominated by our minds. We get to decide what amount of power we will give to our thoughts while meditating. Instead of biting the hooks, we can choose to see them but swim past them. If we swim past them, we protect ourselves from being so impacted by them. Meditation gives us an opportunity to practice seeing the bait and then swimming past it.

It's important to recognize that, in the metaphor, the objective is not to find a spot in the water where there are no baited hooks. On the contrary, the point of the metaphor is that we are all always surrounded by baited hooks. The task we practice in a mindfulness meditation is to find a way to coexist with the bait and the hooks, without biting them. Our task is to practice this within the context of our "hunger." We want to indulge our thoughts. This is why we do it so often. And this is the reason mindfulness meditation is so difficult but is such a valuable tool for taming our minds.

Peace of Mind

This chapter focused on the way meditation can be used to nurture a kinder, gentler presence within you. In other chapters, we will examine the value this more supportive way of being can have for someone preparing to undergo a cosmetic procedure.

When used effectively, meditation can help you live a healthier life. If practiced regularly, it can help you maintain a more peaceful and less reactive mindset. You could more often resist the urge to slavishly respond to every random thought that pops into your mind. This is how meditation "quiets" our mind. It's about diminishing the sense of urgency. And this is how, with practice, meditation can even feel relaxing.

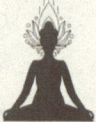

Exercise: Bedtime Loving Sleep Meditation

Reminder: a guided version of this meditation is located at DrAlanGoodwin.com

Instructions: Plan to do this for five minutes or more. Prior to the meditation, read all the instructions below. Please begin by saying these two things aloud or in your mind (if different words feel better to you, use them, but keep the same messages; they're important):

I will begin to sleep now.   I embrace my sleep.

Now, please follow the instructions below.

1. Assume a comfortable position in your bed.

2. Choose a non-defensive posture. Relax your muscles. Uncross arms and legs unless it's uncomfortable.

3. Gently allow your eyes to close.

4. Breathe. Notice your breaths. Pause slightly after the inhale, creating space. From that space, begin a nice, long exhale.

5. Embrace this moment. Feel your self-compassion.

6. Do a body scan, beginning at your feet. Use your breathing to loosen all of your muscles. With every exhale, imagine that you send any tightness out of your body.

7. Notice your breath: the inhales, the space, and the exhales.

8. Slowly repeat this two-part mantra, as many times as needed:

9. Breathe in, feel the space and say *This day is complete.* Then breathe out and say *Complete.*

10. *This day is complete. Complete.*

11. Continuing slow, steady, calm breathing, repeat this new two-part mantra, at least several times:

12. Breathe in, feel the space and say *It's time to rest.* Breathe out and say *I rest.*

13. *It's time to rest. I rest.*

14. Finally, slowly repeat this final two-part mantra, at least several times:

15. Breathe in, feel the space and say *It's time to sleep.* Breathe out and say *I sleep.*

16. *It's time to sleep. I sleep.*

17. As you drift off, repeat any of the mantras you feel would be helpful, as many times as you'd like.

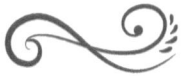

CHAPTER 3

Skin Deeper:
Change Begins Within

*We delight in the beauty of the butterfly, but rarely admit
the changes it has gone through to achieve that beauty.*

— *Maya Angelou*

Uninteresting and Unattractive

"Dude, she's not into me. Seriously, dude, she's not."

I'm going to tell you about twenty-one-year-old Peter in a minute.
For now, I want to use his words to tell you a little about myself.

First, I think it's kind of funny when a client calls me "dude." I also
get a kick out of how gender-neutral "dude" has become. I know that
dates me. That's why I'm telling you this. People under thirty use "dude"
way more liberally than we did when I was under thirty. These days, guys,
girls, and even some psychologists are dudes. I don't like or dislike the

label for myself. I'm just mentioning it to explain that I don't really think the label fits me.

You wouldn't find me in my office in Vans and cargo shorts. I have a friend, Kelli, who cross-dresses a lot. She would label the Vans outfit "dude drag." She likes to say "Everyone has their drag, doll. Everyone." I happen to know some great therapists who dress in dude drag. I just don't. Most days I work in what Kelli calls "therapist drag"—business-casual slacks, a collared or polo shirt, and a wool-blend crew-neck sweater. I'm a roughly middle-aged, Caucasian male with an about average body shape.

I think it's important to describe myself to you because the way I look is always relevant. It's relevant even if I'm working with a client who can't see me. How we appear influences how others treat us. It also influences how we see and treat ourselves. All of this shapes the people we become, including while working.

I aim to be pretty nondescript when I'm at work. This helps keep the focus on the client. I'm trained as a generalist but I work especially well with anxiety disorders. I understand anxiety especially well because I had obsessive-compulsive disorder (OCD) as a young teen. I wasn't diagnosed or treated for OCD as a kid, but I know now that I had it.

I think my own past experience with OCD helps me to empathize with my clients' experiences of struggle and to communicate that to them. As a method of coping, I personally benefit from a meditation practice, and I inform clients of that. I believe this lends credibility when I tell clients that they, too, could benefit from a meditation practice.

So, back to Peter. For a twenty-one-year-old college student, Peter had exceptionally well-defined plans to change himself, both physically and emotionally. "I have my dad's round face, and my mom's short height. The bad skin is probably mainly my own fault from years of being a lazy ass and eating too much chocolate. I've done some research. Once I'm making some money, I'll be able to change all of those things."

This caught me by surprise. Peter hadn't been referred to me for preparation for aesthetic work of any kind. I wasn't expecting him to tell me he wanted to change in those ways. "Oh," I said, "so you plan to undergo some plastic surgery in the future?"

"Yeah, there are lipo procedures that could narrow my face. I'm hoping to do that someday, along with a chin implant. I think those two things could really improve things. And I'd like to get a deep facial peel to fix my acne scars."

Psychologists need to listen carefully to their clients. That may sound obvious, but I mention it now because it requires hearing what a client says and also what a client doesn't say. This was especially relevant in my work with Peter.

Although I had never seen the way Peter got treated out in the world, I felt confident that Peter's opinions of himself didn't match what other people thought of him. I could see that, physically, he was a handsome guy with an athletic physique—built like a football player. And he was a friendly university student. He was in the premed program and was doing well academically.

Unfortunately, when Peter looked at himself, he saw an uninteresting, unattractive guy with a physique that was average at best, and, in his view, actually pudgy. He felt satisfied with his grades but anxious about them because he was convinced he needed to work harder than other students. All other students. He fully expected to encounter academic difficulties in medical school.

Becoming "Better"

Peter, like George, had a tendency to be unkind toward himself. They both also tended to be hard on other people, even if only in their own minds. For both of them, the overactive tendency to criticize contributed to their struggles with depression and anxiety.

Peter sought psychotherapy for the purpose of changing himself into a "better" person. It's common for people to come to me with that intention, and I'll comment on that particular goal again at the end of this chapter.

I was happy to see that Peter's plan was to do the inner work now and commence the plastic surgical procedures when he could afford them. In this chapter, we will discuss the relationship between external (in other words, physical) changes and the internal changes that so often are part of the plan.

It's difficult to achieve growth and change. Change requires reversing course. That's always hard to do. When we choose to make lasting changes, these occur over time and as the result of a process, rather than being the result of a single act. Changes that stand the test of time tend to occur incrementally and as the direct result of focused intentionality and commitment.

Since change is such a complex process, it will be divided into three chapters. This chapter will focus on the internal aspects of the change process. The next chapter will focus on the process of achieving physical changes. And the third will be more general, examining coping strategies that can be applied to the challenges that arise at various stages in the change process.

The Internal Meeting the External: The Talking Face

Let's take a closer look at the change process within the context of cosmetic surgical procedures. Cosmetic procedures are truly profound endeavors. This is especially true of facial procedures. As Ludwig Wittgenstein wrote, "The face is the soul of the body." Our face is central to the emotional and psychological nourishment we receive. We constantly use our face to communicate with the outside world, both in conscious and unconscious ways.

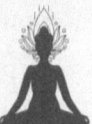

Exercise: The Talking Face

Try this brief exercise. I typically do this with clients who are preparing for a cosmetic facial procedure.

To begin, please think for a minute about a person you know who devotes a healthy amount of attention to self-care. Someone who nurtures their mind and body. Once you find that person, see their face in your mind. Look at it very carefully. Notice their expression. Notice how the muscles in their face help to create that expression. Notice especially their eyes and the corners of their mouth. See what their expression seems to say to you about their thoughts and feelings.

Now take a moment and do the same exercise using a different person. This time, please choose a person you know who tends to neglect their mind and body. We all struggle, but this person compounds their own struggles. Maybe they are a workaholic, or someone who goes through life arguing over unimportant details, or holding grudges, or taking other people's mistakes personally. Focus on this struggling person's face in your mind. Notice their expression. Notice how the muscles in their face help to create their expression. Notice especially their eyes and the corners of their mouth.

Now devote a few minutes to thinking about the impact these two people's faces have on what they receive from the world. Have you noticed how people tend to respond to them? Our faces speak, even before we do. Some people's faces say, "Hello, I'm eager to meet you—and to have you meet me!" Other people's faces say, "I expect you to criticize me and I am prepared to criticize you."

Any intervention that alters a person's face can be very impactful. It's good to appreciate that fact. And it's good to remember that our faces do influence our lived experience.

But these realities refer to what occurs *outside* our bodies and minds. The Talking Face Exercise reminds us that faces are also reflections of what we feel within ourselves. Regardless of the number of facial procedures a person undergoes, somehow that person's inner world will find expression in their face. Nature designed us that way. The face is a tool that our body and mind use to communicate our experience. Although we have some control over what our faces reveal, neither we nor our surgeons have complete control over that. No cosmetic correction, no matter how expertly achieved, can completely erase the effects of an unhappy internal state.

Appearance Change, Inner Transformation, and Kindness

All of this brings us to the real focus of this chapter: the cosmetic patient's internal world. Cosmetic patients often neglect the role their emotional wellness will play in the success of the procedure. Internal and external changes in a person tend to have synergistic relationships with each other. Anytime we seek profound personal growth and change, an inner transformation needs to occur to make the most of the cosmetic changes.

You probably have things you want to change about yourself—appearance, finances, career, or otherwise. Hopefully, you recognize that changes occur as the result of a process. Change occurs over time rather than as a single, sudden event. This means change requires sustained effort and motivation.

When well-intentioned people try to help someone achieve a personal goal, the focus is usually on hard work. The two people look for ways to intensify the person's efforts. "No pain, no gain" often becomes the implicit (or explicit) guiding principle.

There's no doubt diligence and hard work are important elements in the change process. But a vital component that's often ignored is kindness. Hard work is like a whip. Whipping ourselves might motivate us in some moments, but lasting motivation comes more from joy than from fear of pain. When the focus is too much on hard work and not enough on nurturance, burnout is more likely.

One way to nurture ourselves is by bringing more kindness into our lives. When I discuss the issue of kindness with a client seeking personal change, it's typically met with a reaction between indifference and overt rejection.

Kindness is often considered to be at odds with personal growth and change. Change, it is thought, is hard. Kindness is soft. The belief is that the hardness of the change process must be met with the hardness we exhibit when we treat ourselves in unkind and unforgiving ways. No pain, no gain.

Although gender roles are more fluid than in decades past, men are often still socialized to resist vulnerability. Even the mere act of appreciating kindness from other people can feel threatening because of the fear that it might create the impression of neediness and weakness. This resistance to feeling or being perceived as vulnerable sometimes becomes reinforced in the workplace. Of course, women aren't immune to these struggles either, particularly in professions in which aggressiveness is rewarded, such as the legal profession.

I have frequently treated attorneys. As an attorney myself, I know how attorneys sometimes treat one another; I remember experiencing it. Female attorneys often present the same tough-as-nails exterior that many of their male counterparts adopt. I've had female clients who were attorneys. More than once they have explained that their toughness can be a necessary tool for defending against intimidation tactics, particularly by male attorneys. Toughness helps an attorney maintain a distance from the opposing counsel, which is helpful professionally. The problem is, toughness also distances us from our authentic selves. For both men and women, that spiky exoskeleton tends to be hard to take off with your business suit at the end of the day.

The metaphor of the exoskeleton can explain why toughness can be destructive to the cosmetic change process. Sustained motivation requires perseverance during inevitable periods of self-doubt and exhaustion. To conquer our fatigue and fears, we need to understand them. This requires seeing them clearly, with kindness, patience, and curiosity.

The exoskeleton protects a person from being fully seen by others, but it also tends to block the person's view of their authentic self. This inhibits insight, self-respect, and self-compassion. In this way, the tough exoskeleton can diminish self-confidence and motivation.

Peter and Joey

Peter was an adherent to the "tough is best" way of thinking. In addition to the personal assets I already described, Peter was one of the most skilled members of his college soccer team and he was a decorated wrestler. All of this in addition to being an A student majoring in biochemistry.

During one of our sessions, I asked him, "Peter, can you tell me more about your exercise routine? You said you go to the gym. How often?"

"Yeah, I need it. It keeps my vibe positive. I go five or six days a week. I do weights four days a week. I usually do cardio every day I go to the gym unless I did it at practice."

I had a feeling there might be helpful information contained in the way Peter used his workouts. "Help me get a sense of what your workout is like," I said. "When you lift weights, do you use a partner or do you work out alone?"

"I definitely lift alone. I'm better at motivating myself."

"Okay, that's helpful. Can you give me an example of how you motivate yourself?"

After a pause, Peter laughed and looked away, shifting in his chair. When he looked back at me, he said, "I didn't expect you to ask that. I can answer it, but you're gonna think it's weird."

"Try me." I smiled.

"I'll need to explain. Okay, so, if I'm lifting a lot, I call myself 'Joey.' I say 'Come on, Joey. Do it, Joey.' I say it to myself just like that."

Peter said it with a kind of ominous tone. He sounded like a bully threatening someone. His voice held an implicit warning, like, "If you don't do this, Joey, there's gonna be trouble." I called it to Peter's attention.

Peter smiled sheepishly. "Yeah, well, that's kind of exactly what it is. Joey was a kid in my neighborhood when I was, like, nine until I was about fourteen. Then he got homeschooled and we hardly ever saw him anymore. Nobody liked him. He was one of those kids who whined any time he didn't get his way. So, we'd pick on him. It wasn't really cool of us, but he deserved it, to be honest."

"Hmm, okay," I said, still confused, "and you say Joey's name when you're trying to lift heavy weights?"

"It's kind of convoluted, I guess. See, when I say that to myself, what I'm really saying is, like, come on, don't be like Joey. Like, 'Are you gonna be a baby? Don't be a Joey!' See?" Then Peter turned to me and said, "You're gonna tell me it's not cool that I say that to myself, aren't you?"

That was a loaded question. In traditional psychotherapy, the therapist is mostly silent and avoids answering questions directly. The solution-focused psychotherapy I provide is different. It's often helpful for me to give direct answers—but not always. This was one of the latter situations.

"Peter, can I promise to answer that after you give me a few more words that describe how you think of Joey? I just want to understand this better."

"Oh, that's easy. Weak, pitiful, incapable, immature, disgusting, nauseating. Did I say weak?" Peter laughed. "How am I doing? Need some more?"

"Nope, that'll do it. I think I have a vague idea how you still feel about Joey."

He laughed, and I smiled.

Peter guessed right. How he spoke about Joey did seem unhealthy to me, on multiple levels. I felt sad for Joey, of course, but Joey wasn't my client. My responsibility was to help Peter. My concern was the self-destructive impact on Peter of this way of essentially threatening himself.

I knew I needed to be careful in addressing this issue with him. When a coping method is working for a client, it's important to respect that. It's good to integrate coping methods that have worked for the client into their self-care and treatment program. And yet it's also important to be honest with the client. The truth was Peter's method was going to be difficult for me to embrace.

Peter was coming to me for help achieving personal growth and change. He believed his surgery would improve his self-confidence, but he correctly recognized that there was psychological work he needed to do as well.

Peter had a self-destructive tendency to maintain ugly and judgmental thoughts about himself. It wasn't a coincidence that he also still ridiculed poor Joey, even if only in his mind. We needed to process how Peter's abusive way of treating Joey informed the way he treated himself.

"Listen," I said, "I should be clear about something: I don't believe my job is to make you into a different person. In fact, I think my first job is to respect you and to honor the behaviors and thoughts that seem to work for you."

"Okay," Peter said, "but still, you're not happy with how I use that 'Joey' label, are you?"

"To be honest, no, I'm not. My concern is this: what happens when one day you aren't able to perform at something as well as you want to? It sounds like the consequence will be that you'll think of yourself like a version of Joey."

"Well, yeah, that's the point," Peter replied.

"I understand. The thing is, the possibility that you could see yourself as a weak person, as someone who embodies the characteristics you associate with and reject in Joey, creates a sort of weapon in your mind. And it seems to me it's like you're holding that weapon up to your nose and you are always ready to hit yourself with it if you decide you deserve it. It threatens you. *You* threaten you, Peter. That's my concern: that you're always one poor performance away from feeling weak, pitiful, incapable, and so on. You see what I mean?"

"Well, I guess so. But still, it works," Peter said. "I'm not sure I want to let go of it."

"That's alright. You don't have to let go of it. I just want you to start examining these ways of being that you've developed over the years. And on the subject of Joey, I think it'll be good for us to consider examining your feelings about the idea of being like Joey."

At this moment, Peter removed his tough exoskeleton. His mood seemed to become much more somber. He paused a while without speaking. Then he said, "I've always hated Joey's weakness. Being like Joey actually scares me. I feel afraid when I think about it. The thing is, in a way, I kind of already feel like him sometimes. Definitely when I'm around girls."

"You feel that way because you expect them to reject you?"

"Yeah," Peter said, "I do. I expect it and it always happens."

"As you talk about this now, you sound like you're aware of the ways Joey must have struggled."

"I guess that's true, but I hate that. I hate the idea of being anything like Joey. I hate relating to him in any way."

"I can see your dilemma," I said. "You want to dislike him and disrespect him because you see him as pathetic and incapable. And yet you're aware that the same part of you that condemns weakness in him and in other people also condemns it in yourself."

"Well, I do. But I don't see what healthy alternative there is. If I'm honest about it, he was a loser. He's never gonna be happy. I don't want a life like that."

"I'm glad to hear you want to be happy in life, Peter. I want that for you too. I think the solution to your dilemma lies in seeing people's struggles differently. I think we need to challenge this habit you've developed of being so condemning of failure. I guess I'm saying that I'm glad you want to win in life, but I want to help you to be prepared for the times when you won't win. Because loss is a part of life, too. More importantly, loss is often what spurs the most growth."

Peter sat in silence. He avoided my efforts to make eye contact. He seemed to be deep in thought, and he appeared agitated. His hands cupped his kneecaps as his knees rose and fell rapidly. His entire body was in motion. His lips were tensed and he was shaking his head as if repeating the word "no" in his mind. Finally, he looked up and made eye contact with me. As he spoke, his words seemed measured and his tone was tense: "I mean, that sounds nice," he said, "but, to be honest, it just doesn't sound like much of a plan for success. It sounds more like a recipe for wallowing in self-pity and ignoring incompetence in people." And with that, he slipped back into the exoskeleton. But that was okay.

He'd had the experience of taking it off, even if only briefly. That would make it easier for him to do it again.

I was happy Peter was willing to respond so honestly. It was helpful to hear how committed he felt to these ways of thinking and being. I told him that and added, "Peter, I do hope you'll try to remain open to the possibility that seeing other people's struggles in a way that helps you relate to them might have the opposite effect on you that wallowing would have. That it might, in fact, even empower you."

Surgical Self-Sabotage by Demanding Too Much

Peter's style of self-motivation isn't only found in young men. Rigidity and abusiveness seem to be more common than ever, and are directed both at the self and others. The struggles of life often lead people to behave in demanding, impatient, and judgmental ways in order to feel resilient.

I suppose this can be linked to the "no pain, no gain" credo. Whatever the origin, I do find most clients seeking growth and change resist the idea of using self-care and kindness to tap into their strengths.

Rigidity and impatience have particular relevance for patients seeking cosmetic changes. When these patients retain unrealistic goals and insist on quick results that ignore their body's need to heal, they often behave in ways that sabotage the outcome. Despite surgeons reminding them that every human body is unique and needs time to recover from the trauma of a procedure, patients sometimes want the desired outcome to reveal itself too soon after the procedure. Attaching an unreasonable demand onto the change process at best handicaps the process, and at worst completely derails it, causing the person to feel like a failure, which can give rise to its own series of consequences.

This is why, for some cosmetic surgery patients, it's so important to engage in effective, introspective psychotherapy prior to the procedure.

Some patients rightly point to goals they reached in life because of their demanding way of being. The problem is, in the realm of cosmetic procedures, complete predictability is never achievable. As a result, rigid outcome demands often lead to disappointment. Prior to the intervention itself, psychotherapy can help a patient become more aware of their tendency toward rigidity and of the impact it can have on the success of a cosmetic procedure.

Peter, for instance, had devoted years to critically examining his facial features. People like Peter invest so much time and energy in criticizing themselves that it becomes a reflexive way of being.

Those excessive demands have a way of catching up with us. Overly demanding people are difficult to please and therefore often struggle with chronic bouts of unhappiness. If Peter were to change the way he looked without lessening his tendency to be so self-critical, there would be a higher likelihood that he would be dissatisfied with any outcome.

I worked with Peter for several years. That fact alone reveals a lot about Peter. He was committed to carefully and honestly examining himself in psychotherapy. He worked hard with me. Over time, he did relinquish what we came to call "The Joey Method."

Peter utilized various tools in his psychotherapy, including journaling. He did exercises like one for transforming negative self-talk that is reproduced at the end of this chapter. That exercise helps a person quiet the critical part of their mind and raise the volume of the complimentary and hopeful part. He also became a daily mindfulness meditator. Consistent with the burgeoning body of research on this subject, Peter found mindfulness meditation helped him slow down his reflexive tendency to be overly critical of himself and other people. In time, he developed more self-compassion and patience.

Mainly, Peter was able to see the link between his own self-esteem issues and the demanding way he tended to look at himself and the world.

He also came to realize that his habit of engaging in judgmental and critical self-talk tended to preserve and reinforce a sense of personal inadequacy. It fueled a persistent and unhealthy need to *un-prove* his own inadequacy to himself. In the long run, he felt empowered when he was able to eliminate from consideration the idea that he might one day decide to think of himself as a complete loser.

Anxiety, Low Self-Esteem, and Habitual Self-Sabotage

Peter and I also focused on his struggles with anxiety. The way he raised the issue was in reference to his never asking women out on dates. He believed he *knew* most weren't interested in him. His only dating experiences had occurred when the woman initiated the idea. There were two of these incidents, each involving women with whom he had worked on a class project.

You may recall that Peter intended to undergo procedures to narrow his face, alter his chin, and correct acne scarring. Peter explained he chose those procedures because he believed he wasn't attractive enough. He was still considering a rhinoplasty procedure and also one to enhance the squareness of his jawline, but planned to wait and see if those were necessary after the other procedures.

To assist our discussion of his perceived undesirability to women, I administered a brief tool that I've reproduced at the end of this chapter. The tool is called the Appearance Self-Consciousness Measure (ASM). This simple screening tool does what its title suggests: it gives the client and me a sense of how self-conscious they are about their attractiveness. Not surprisingly, Peter endorsed a number of items that indicated he struggled with self-consciousness about his attractiveness.

"So, you probably realize that your score indicates you're pretty self-conscious about your attractiveness," I said.

"Yeah, I could have told you that." He smiled. "But honestly, I don't think I'm being overly critical of myself. I think I'm just being honest. Most girls aren't interested in dating me. I've seen it."

"I believe you were answering honestly. The thing is, I'm not convinced it's accurate. Over time, I just hope you'll be open to exploring the things that led you to draw that conclusion."

Like a lot of people who score high on the ASM, Peter's view of himself didn't seem to match the objective truth on some issues. For instance, the way women treated him: he was approached by women fairly often. When I asked him about this, he explained that he believed they liked his friendship but wouldn't be interested in dating him. But he never dared to test that assumption.

Peter had some self-sabotaging tendencies that we were able to address in his psychotherapy. His treatment is relevant to many cosmetic procedure patients because of his tendency to be so demanding of himself and of others. Like a lot of cosmetic patients, Peter pursued goals with passion and without apology. That attitude can arise out of an achievement-oriented focus on one's goals. Unfortunately, in cosmetic procedure patients, this kind of passion is often expressed in self-destructive ways.

Peter's rigid demands were often fueled by inaccurate and excessively critical views of aspects of his appearance. When self-criticisms involve personal and subjective issues such as one's beauty, cosmetic procedures are less likely to eliminate them to the person's satisfaction. The reasons for this and the ways to overcome this tendency will be discussed in more detail in several parts of the book. For now, the important point is Peter's physical flaws became a tormenting enemy, glaring back at him through mirrors on a daily basis. Surgical procedures can change the image in the mirror, but they can't change the perception of the viewer. That's what psychotherapy is for.

Shame, Guilt, Self-Talk, and Change

A book like this that is aimed at helping people maintain emotional wellness can't achieve its objective without addressing the abusive impact of overly critical self-talk. Self-talk is a term that refers to a person's inner dialogue. Over the years, I've heard so many ugly things that people have said to themselves, wrongly believing that self-criticisms and even self-mockery would motivate them to achieve growth and change. I've found people often use the same phrases on themselves repeatedly. Sometimes the messages can be so vivid and powerful that patients and even mental health professionals label them "voices" and mistake them for symptoms of psychosis. Usually self-talk is not psychosis; it's just a powerful form of self-abuse.

Negative self-talk is common. The frequency and intensity of it typically increases during personal struggles. For instance, if a person fails to achieve something, their inner dialogue might be, "You're such a loser," or "You're an idiot," or "I hate you," or "I hate myself." Another common habit is to repeat phrases other people have said to them, like "What's the matter with you?" or "How could you be so stupid?" In more severe and dangerous cases, the client might say things like "You should die" or "I hate my life."

These phrases may sound different from Peter's "Come on, Joey!", but in fact they all reveal the same core problem. These kinds of critical internal messages reinforce feelings of inadequacy. In this way, they undermine our self-confidence.

Many people have an active critical inner voice. One reason for this is the widespread belief that shame is an effective tool for growth and change. The belief is that if we just shame ourselves intensely enough, we will create the changes we seek. Again, a form of "no pain, no gain."

In reality, self-shaming often has the opposite impact. Shame has been defined as a core sense of inadequacy. Shame involves a deeper injury than guilt. Guilt refers to the belief that we have misbehaved. Shame refers not merely to doing a bad act, but rather to a person's deep-seated fundamental inadequacy.

The difference between shame and guilt is that guilt can be addressed, such as with an apology. Shame cannot be eliminated with a mere apology. With shame, failure seems to confirm the person's inadequacy. This is why shame often fuels procrastination and underachievement. Shame is so overwhelmingly painful that it causes people who struggle with it to feel paralyzed, unable to tolerate the risk of failure.

The most destructive aspect of shame is that it impairs future achievements. When we communicate shaming phrases to ourselves, they seem to speak not only of how we just performed, but also of how we expect to perform. So, these phrases encourage us to wrongly assume that if we failed in the past, we will fail in the future. This diminishes our confidence and our sense of hopefulness.

The good news is we can identify feelings of shame and alter them. Effective psychotherapy directly targets the unsupportive ways you treat yourself. Over time, you can reprogram your mind, eliminating unhealthy ways of speaking to and about yourself. The result is improved motivation and lower levels of depression and hopelessness.

This is a nice time to bring this discussion full circle by referencing something Peter said. I noted earlier that Peter sought psychotherapy to become a "better person." Effective psychotherapy helps us recognize that our humanity presupposes flaws. If we can accept that humans are flawed, we move a step closer to developing the ability to treat ourselves and others with more kindness.

Being Human

This chapter focused on the value of finding ways to embrace your humanity. All of us perform poorly sometimes. We all make mistakes—repeatedly.

Effective psychotherapy helps us embrace these as characteristics of being human rather than as symptoms of inadequacy. When we humanize ourselves, we empower ourselves.

The act of humanizing one's self has particular relevance for coping with cosmetic procedures. When a patient replaces rigid demands with compassion and forgiveness, the patient creates space for embracing a broader variety of surgical outcomes. The shift away from demands helps the patient to honor not only the outcomes of their efforts but also the processes leading to the outcomes and the intentions underlying their actions. People who do this are more likely to feel gratitude more often and disappointment less often both in cosmetic procedures and in life.

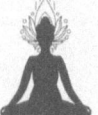

Exercise: Converting Negative Self-Talk into Positive Self-Talk

Let's now examine an exercise to reduce overly critical self-talk. In my experience, people who commit to doing this at least several times each week begin to change their mindset. The people closest to you will also see changes, including in how you respond to them.

At the end of every day (most people like to choose about an hour before bedtime), sit with a pen and your journal (or your computer, if you are using that). Draw a table with four columns. From left to right, label your columns Situation, Negative Self-Talk, Positive Self-Talk, and Alternative Positive Self-Talk (See below).

Situation	Negative Self-Talk	Positive Self-Talk	Alternative Positive Self-Talk

Now think back on your day. Think of a challenging moment you faced. For this exercise, the moment will be considered a "situation." Place at least one situation in the left column. Now close your eyes and sit quietly for a minute or two. Breathe normally and focus on just being present with the situation you have chosen to focus on.

As you recall the situation, try to get in touch with the feelings you felt in that moment. Use the information about those feelings to recall unkind messages you said to yourself. Whenever you feel ready, begin to write those messages down in the Negative Self-Talk column. List any such message you can recall. Remember, the messages can be explicit ("Why am I so stupid?" or "I hate my cheeks") or implicit ("I recall that I thought I was ugly," or "I thought I was inferior").

Now return to your breath and, if you'd like, close your eyes again. Focus again on the situation. This time, try to recall any supportive self-statements. When you feel ready, return to your journal and, in the column labeled positive self-statements, list all of those that you can recall.

Once you have completed the first three columns, examine them. If you listed more than one situation, examine one situation at a time. Look at each situation and then look at what you said to yourself about it. Notice how many critical self-statements you recalled compared to the number of supportive ones. Also, notice whether each critical self-statement is addressed, even if indirectly, in an encouraging one. For instance, if there is a self-statement "I always sound like an idiot," see whether there is a supportive self-statement that counterbalances that, such as "It was thoughtful of me to speak up" or "I had good intentions," or "Everyone makes mistakes sometimes, or "Doing something poorly doesn't make me an idiot," or "I have plenty of abilities that confirm I'm not stupid." Draw a line from any negative self-statement to a positive one that counterbalances it, if there is one.

The purpose of the last column is to make sure there is at least one supportive self-statement to counter each negative self-statement. If you find a negative self-statement that was not counter-balanced by a positive self-statement, create a positive self-statement and draw a line that connects it to the negative self-statement that it counter-balances. If you already created affirming alternative statements for every negative self-statement, that's great. You can stop, or you can create other kind, self-compassionate, and accurate self-statements that counter the negative self-statements.

Creating more positive self-statements is a healthy exercise in and of itself. It's good practice. It would be a great idea to write the positive self-statements down on an index card that you carry around with you or enter them into the notes section in your phone. You can then pull them out and use them as mantras at various times during the day. This is a great way to acquire a more positive, self-affirming, and success-oriented mindset.

Sample table:

Situation	Negative Self-Talk	Positive Self-Talk	Alternative Positive Self-Talk
Seeing Judy at the café and recommending the mocha coffee.	Your stupid brain! You know Judy is dieting!	It was an instant and you forgot about her diet. You're human.	
	How could you be so insensitive?	You're human.	
	You're still so selfish!	⟶	You often think of others.
	Mind your own business—for once!	⟶	You were just being friendly.

One more thing: remember that this is a cognitive exercise. The objective with the last column is accuracy, not blind positivity. So, we don't want to counterbalance a condemning comment such as "I'm a total idiot" with the equally inaccurate "I'm the smartest person on the planet." Examples of good alternative self-statements are listed above. Others would be "Breathe. No one is perfect," or "You are growing. It's just a mistake," or "Honor your humanity," or "One moment doesn't define you," or "You're doing fine," or "It's okay to not know something or to misspeak sometimes." Do you notice a pattern? The positive self-statements are examples of things a friend might say to you. Although you can use the statements listed above, it's a good exercise to create some on your own. The ones you create for yourself often have more of an impact on how you feel and on how you treat yourself.

This exercise gets you into the habit of being more kind, balanced, and reasonable in your thoughts about yourself and your performance. So, try to be mindful as you do the exercise. Notice what the exercise is teaching you about the things you say to yourself and about how you treat yourself. Use that knowledge to begin to notice these habits throughout each day. When you notice them, take a moment to alter negative self-talk so that it is positive and affirming. Doing this will absolutely help you to improve the way you think about yourself. And that will benefit you in literally every part of your life.

Final note: Have patience with yourself. It takes years for us to acquire the habits of treating ourselves in certain ways. You will not change those habits overnight. By consistently focusing on these thinking habits, you will be able to change them. It begins with one thought.

 Appearance Self-Consciousness Measure (ASM)

Imagine experiencing each of the events described below. For each one, use the following scale to rate how intensely you feel self-conscious about your appearance, when the experience occurs:

Scoring

0 = It never causes me to feel self-conscious

1 = I feel somewhat distracted by it

2 = I feel completely consumed in my own self-conscious thoughts whenever this happens:

1. When I see an image of myself (photo, video, or mirror).

2. When I weigh myself.

3. When I'm at cafes, parks, or other public venues where people see me.

4. When I'm engaged in a sport requiring movement.

5. When I notice an attractive person.

6. When someone makes any comment about my appearance.

7. After I have finished eating something.

8. When I am with someone I am interested in romantically.

9. When I eat something in public.

Scoring this screening tool is easy. Any item that is rated a 2 is an indication of a potentially serious problem that should be discussed with a mental health professional. If you have three or more items endorsed with a 1, you have indicated you are distracted by your appearance in several different circumstances, and you really should consider speaking with a mental health professional to assess whether you are overly concerned about your appearance. Although items you rated a 1 are not necessarily indicative of an unhealthy preoccupation with your attractiveness, discussing any of those items with a mental health professional would likely be illuminating. If you rated each item zero, your responses suggest you don't struggle in the same ways many people who tend to be overly self-conscious struggle.

Exercise: My Change Process: A Journaling Exercise

In this chapter, we began looking at the process of change. The more you can apply the contents of this book to your own life, the more helpful it will be to you. It seems fitting, then, to end the chapter with an exercise that helps you explore your own process. To do that, I suggest you continue the journaling process you began after Chapter 1.

The Hope and Change exercise at the end of Chapter 1 helped you begin to examine your thoughts and feelings connected to this cosmetic procedure. This next exercise is called the My Change Process journaling exercise. This exercise can be used in several ways. First, it's a self-diagnostic tool that helps you continue to identify and clarify the hopes, fears, and expectations you are bringing to this process.

Another function of this exercise is it gives you rich information that you can bring to a mental health professional. The questions are designed to address subjects that often have relevance for people when they consider cosmetic interventions.

Use your journal to discuss your reactions to each item. If some items seem less relevant to you, it's fine to devote less time to them, but do notice them. You might take a moment to acknowledge when an issue is not one with which you struggle, because it's helpful to acknowledge your strengths. You might also choose to describe specifically why you do *not* fear certain undesired outcomes listed in the exercise.

As with all the exercises in this book, I recommend that you take your time completing it. Try not to rush through it. Also, try to complete the exercises in an environment where you are able to think. Honoring your preparatory processes will enhance the value and relevance they have for you.

Please begin by envisioning your planned cosmetic work. There is no way to know precisely what changes it will, or will not, create. The following statements are intended to help you identify your current fears and hopes, plus new ones that could arise. Try to allow yourself to write about everything that comes to mind.

After the procedure,

1. I hope my friendships will change in these ways:

2. I hope my social habits will change in these ways:

3. I hope my romantic life will change in these ways:

    a. How and why do I see this change occurring in my love life?

    b. How do I hope my romantic partner(s) will treat me differently?

4. I hope the clothes I wear will change in these ways:

5. I hope my family will treat me differently in these ways:

6. I hope my experience at work or school will change in these ways:

7. I hope my hobbies will change in these ways:

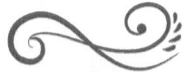

CHAPTER 4

Lifted: Changing the Outside

Every man over forty is responsible for his face.

—*Abraham Lincoln*

Anyone in Her Right Mind

Remember Jayne, from Chapter 1? Jayne was the tough-minded sixty-eight-year-old "Bea Arthur type" who was preparing for a facial procedure. She was also confronting her own judgments about these sorts of changes.

As I begin to talk about Jayne, I think it will be helpful to share some information about psychotherapy. Psychotherapy should never be serving the therapist's personal needs. The whole point of therapy is that it is the only relationship we ever have in which we don't have to give anything in return for what we receive. The only thing the psychotherapist is entitled to is their fee. A client doesn't owe a therapist politeness, directness, tact, impeccable hygiene, or even honesty. Psychotherapy is most beneficial when the client feels free to allow their true self to emerge rather than presenting a version they think will please their therapist.

I share this information with you because I think it will help you to consider and clarify how you might use psychotherapy. It also gives me an opportunity to admit something: the reality is that skilled psychotherapists do derive much more from their work than income. Most of us really value and enjoy our work, and we like the clients we serve. It gives us pleasure to engage with them. I always feel compassion and admiration for my clients' courage. Always. I always feel privileged to be trusted and to be included in their growth process. And I do feel a sense of achievement and, yes, even affirmation from my work. So, I do benefit personally in many ways.

This is especially relevant here, because Jayne was a delight to help. Don't get me wrong, she was tough and challenging. But it was always a pleasure to sit with her. You might have guessed that when you read my description of her; after all, what gay male of a certain age would not like and admire "a Bea Arthur type"? Okay, back to Bea—I mean Jayne.

"There is a part of myself," she explained during our initial session, "that thinks anyone in their right mind would ask me what the hell has come over me to be considering this? This is *not* me. I've always advocated for women to fully embrace their age. That part of me still wonders why people like you are not talking me out of this."

"Are you asking me to do that for you?" I asked.

Jayne laughed and, without hesitation, replied, "Oh, no, sweetie. Trust me, if I thought you didn't know better than to try that, I wouldn't be here. And I know better than to ask you to do that for me. No, this is something that only I can resolve. I need to examine why I have these doubts. But I'd like you to help me do that."

Jayne had explored her cosmetic options carefully. By the time she was referred to me, she had already decided which procedure she would choose if she were to go through with it. She chose several distinct surgical interventions, all intended to reverse signs of aging and to eliminate what Jayne called "my resting bitch face."

Jayne gave me permission to speak with her cosmetic surgeon. He explained he referred her to me for psychotherapy because he was concerned that her sadness and anger might undermine the success of the procedure. He had known Jayne socially for years, and he saw the changes in her in recent months. He said her typical good-natured sarcasm had given way to darker qualities. She had become irritable and cynical. He sensed a deep sadness in Jayne, particularly because he knew of the recent life experiences she had endured.

Jayne's surgeon was psychologically sophisticated. He'd been referring patients to me for a number of years. He knew Jayne was in the throes of a traumatic post-divorce period. Due to the events that led to the divorce, she found herself much more inclined to see the darkness in the world than the light.

Jayne's Path

Jayne's path to cosmetic surgery began in earnest about twelve months prior to the procedure. That was around the time when, out of the blue, her husband of thirty-eight years announced he wanted a divorce. To make matters immeasurably worse, Jayne soon learned that, about a year prior to his announcement, he had begun a secret romance with Jayne's best friend. Her former best friend and her ex-husband got married days after Jayne's divorce was finalized, leaving Jayne traumatized by a sense of betrayal and abandonment.

Like most people who met her, I found Jayne very impressive. She had a sharp, clear mind. She was on top of things, keenly aware and observant. Tall, with a relatively low voice, she had a penchant for coming up with clever quips, which she delivered deadpan. She was very funny and was always impeccably dressed.

Jayne and I discussed her objectives for the surgical procedures. She explained she was only indirectly interested in age reversal: "I worked in Los Angeles in the fashion and entertainment industry for many years. It's a tough industry. You need to know yourself or they'll eat you alive. I'm not a young woman, so I don't expect people to see me as one. I feel sad for those older women who seem forever trapped in their need to look thirty-five. That's not me. My focus is on achieving a particular aesthetic. My objective has very little to do with youth and nothing to do with desperation."

I thought it was important to interject at this point. "That's a very particular word, desperation. Can you say more about that?"

Jayne paused. She shifted in her seat and focused directly on me, holding her gaze on me for a few beats for emphasis before replying. "Let me tell you something, there is not a desperate bone in my body. There are furious bones. There are vengeful bones. I admit that. But there are no desperate bones. I'd never give them the satisfaction of feeling desperation."

Comments like this suggested it might be difficult to convince Jayne to allow self-compassion and kindness to guide her. She was like Peter in that way.

"I wouldn't want to encourage you to feel desperation," I said. "But I see your tenderness. It's hidden, but I see it. I wonder when you intentionally allow your tenderness to be seen."

"I think tenderness is fine for other people," she explained, "but I'm not a big fan of vulnerability. It's just not my style. Sometimes you have to take things like a ma—" Jayne stopped before saying "man." She shifted in the armchair, breathed in and out once, seemed to compose herself, and then continued, "like an adult. Sometimes there's just no easy way out, no soft landing."

Jayne was going through the darkest time of her life. I needed to honor her self-protectiveness. I needed to strike a balance between pushing her to explore her vulnerability and respecting her need to maintain her sense of safety and emotional stability.

I recognized that if I was going to sell Jayne on the value of kindness and self-compassion, the payoff was going to have to be something other than vulnerability.

Fortunately, there is a different payoff, and it's the opposite of vulnerability. Jayne had always embraced high standards. I knew she would appreciate any work we did if the objective was excellence.

Jayne needed to recognize that, in her situation, kindness and self-compassion were intimately tied to excellence. One aspect of excellence can be thought of as her postsurgery mindset. In other words, as we discussed regarding Peter, Jayne's rigid standards could cause her to enter the procedure with an overly narrow and uncompromising definition of a successful outcome. Cosmetic surgery outcomes are never entirely predictable. One way Jayne could behave with more self-compassion would be for her to embrace that reality.

For anyone, but especially for Jayne, accepting a less-than-perfect outcome would have been much easier said than done. There was a lot riding on this procedure. It represented a restarting of her life. She felt as though the cosmetic changes would enable her to regain her identity. That's a tall order for a surgical procedure. This is what I hoped to help her explore in psychotherapy.

Cosmetic Change as a Means of Regaining Control of Your Future

During the year-long divorce process, Jayne struggled with an enormous amount of sadness and anger. She experienced a near-constant stream of negative thoughts and feelings, and she felt convinced they had altered her face. "Faces tell stories," Jayne explained. "I know that's true, but I resent it. My story is none of anyone's fucking business. I don't need to have it written all over my face."

Jayne wanted to regain a softer, more energetic, and more hopeful physical presentation. "Regain" is the operative term. Her goals were very much linked to the divorce, in Jayne's mind. "I want to stop seeing my ex-husband and my former friend every time I look at my face. For fourteen months, I've been wearing the face *they* gave me. I'm sick and tired of that. I want *my* face back."

When we discussed her history, Jayne explained she was never a fan of cosmetic procedures. She had felt self-conscious about her eyes throughout her adult life, but she had always resisted the temptation to have them "fixed." Essentially, she explained that her eyes had an intensity that was considered not feminine enough.

In her twenties and thirties she had been employed both as an on-camera spokesperson and as a makeup artist. I've continually been reminded by people involved in the entertainment business of how harsh it can be. Jayne recalled being reminded of her "eye issues" many times. She saw them and other people told her about them. Her skill and knowledge enabled her to become adept at using makeup to accentuate the attractive intensity in her eyes while not causing herself to appear masculine, intimidating, or unfriendly.

"So, Jayne, you were self-conscious about your eyes, but you never considered consulting a plastic surgeon before now?"

"Oh no. No way. Do you know how many people I've seen ruin their faces by having work done on their eyes? One bad eye job ruins a face. But now I really need it. And I've looked at this surgeon's work. He does beautiful work. His work isn't noticeable. That's exactly what I want."

Jayne explained that, in the youth-centered entertainment business, she had gradually become more self-conscious about her appearance. On-camera work dried up for her as she entered her forties. The impact of that was minimal, though, because her intellect and drive enabled her to successfully transition into a producer role.

She never felt compelled to undergo a cosmetic medical procedure. After all, she no longer did on-camera work. And besides, she had an active career and she felt loved by her husband.

Then came the betrayals, and the divorce. Her ex-husband's behavior injured her very deeply. It prompted her to reassess a lot of truths she thought she knew. Her best friend's betrayal also weighed heavily on her.

Jayne explained, "Many times, I've looked back at my calendar and focused on days when I was unaware of the affair. I've looked back and recalled the events and the conversations over lunch or cocktails on one of the many days I met my former friend. I've tried to recall the ways she spoke to me. She was deceiving me during every minute of every one of those occasions." Jayne paused, focusing intently. When she continued her tone was quieter, more pensive and searching. "That's been so hard to let go of. How does a person *do* that? What *kind* of a person does that? And I wonder…I wonder how I could have been so blind. Me, of all people. How did I not see it? How did I not see who she really was?"

The process of reconciling herself with the past, and of adjusting to her new life, led Jayne to reevaluate what she wanted out of life. She decided she was not finished exploring life and finding love and joy. This is what led her to rethink her decision regarding cosmetic surgery.

"One day I was looking into the mirror at the new, deeper wrinkles that had developed on my forehead and at the corners of my mouth. I felt the strangest feeling. The next thing I knew, I felt almost faint. My breath felt constricted, and I suddenly felt trapped. That's the only way I can describe it. I didn't know what was happening. I don't have any health issues, knock wood. It didn't make any sense. So, I went to the kitchen and made myself a cup of tea, and I just sat quietly for a few minutes. That was when I had an epiphany: I think I feel trapped by these changes in my body. Looking back, that was when I began seriously considering surgery."

Jayne felt trapped not only by her own feelings about her appearance, but also by her perception of how others had begun to view her. After the divorce, she said she felt exposed and evaluated. "I felt I had acquired a kind of transparency. I felt judged by some people and pitied by others. I didn't ask for either of those. Pity is the worst form of judgment, if you ask me. How disrespectful! I so resented it. I got it from colleagues and also from the people I supervised. They all meant well, but I just wished they'd all...I just wanted them to mind their own business. I wanted to be left alone. But I could not get away from it."

"You felt as though they were reacting to your appearance?" I asked. "That the way you looked led them to treat you differently?"

"Yes," Jayne said. "I think it was, quite literally, written all over my face. I wanted to get a fresh start, but I felt that my face announced too much of the past year. I had lost control over what my face communicated. I wanted that control back."

Cosmetic Change for Personal Growth

When Jayne first contacted me, she was concerned I would judge her. There were good reasons for her to feel concerned. It's not uncommon for people like Jayne to be treated as though her objectives were unhealthy. I've had a number of patients like Jayne: women older than sixty-five who reported they felt pressured to avoid cosmetic surgery. Some people presume those procedures are all symptomatic of the way society oppresses and objectifies women. The older female patients are viewed as victims. This shaming set of presumptions often leads patients to resist speaking openly about it, even to therapists.

The reality is often starkly different from the presumptions. From the perspective of industry leaders like Jayne, cosmetic work can provide an opportunity to feel more in control over important aspects not only of their personal but also their professional lives. In particular, these patients often report they are not ready to retire and the workplace is a very ageist place. A successful cosmetic intervention can extend a person's professional viability by decades.

In fact, there is psychological research that supports the notion that these physical changes can have profound impacts on the way patients feel about themselves. A modest study in 2008 involved ninety-three patients who underwent a rhinoplasty or a "surgery for the aging face."[1] This study found levels of self-consciousness about one's appearance decreased after cosmetic facial surgeries. Similar findings were reported in a 2009 UK study.[2] In the UK study, cosmetic surgical patients exhibited multiple psychological improvements after their procedures. Improvements included reduced levels of depression, anxiety, and self-consciousness about the aspect of themselves that had been surgically altered.

Naturally, improvements in a person's psychological well-being often also positively impact other areas of their life such as performance in

1 Litner, Jason A., Rotenberg, Brian W., Dennis, Maureen, and Adamson, Peter A. (Mar. 2008). *Impact of Cosmetic Facial Surgery on Satisfaction With Appearance and Quality of Life*, Archives of Facial Plastic Surgery, 10(2), pp.79-83.

2 Timothy P. Moss & David L. Harris (2009). Psychological change after aesthetic plastic surgery: A prospective controlled outcome study, *Psychology, Health & Medicine*, 14(5), 567-572, DOI: 10.1080/13548500903112374.

social and work settings. Though such changes are impressive, one might question how robust these benefits tend to be. A 2008 study[3] examined one hundred cosmetic surgery patients beginning at three months after the surgical procedure and continuing until two years after the procedure. Patients were assessed using measures of self-esteem, body image, and depressive symptoms. The study found that most patients did acquire an improved body image, less self-consciousness, and more of a sense of attractiveness. Patients' reports of positive feelings persisted twenty-four months after the surgical procedure.

Some research has specifically examined whether these sorts of personal gains are also reflected in professional success. A study conducted in 2013 examined the impact of a cosmetic procedure on a patient's psychological well-being,[4] comparing patients who underwent a procedure with those who were interested in undergoing one but who did not go through with it. The study found lower postsurgical levels of anxiety, social phobia, depression, and body dysmorphia in the people who had the procedures compared to those who did not. Of more direct relevance to professional success, this study also found those who had the procedure experienced increases in goal attainment, quality of life, life satisfaction, attractiveness, mental and physical health, well-being, self-efficacy, and self-esteem.

---

3 David B. Sarwer, PhD, Alison L. Infield, James L. Baker, MD, Laurie A. Casas, MD, Paul M. Glat, MD, Alan H. Gold, MD, Mark L. Jewell, MD, Don LaRossa, MD, Foad Nahai, MD, V. Leroy Young, MD. (May 2008). Two-Year Results of a Prospective, Multi-Site Investigation of Patient Satisfaction and Psychosocial Status Following Cosmetic Surgery, *Aesthetic Surgery Journal*, 28(3), pp.245–250, https://doi.org/10.1016/j.asj.2008.02.003.

4 Margraf, J., Meyer. A.H., Lavallee, K.L. (2013). Well-Being From the Knife? Psychological Effects of Aesthetic Surgery. *Clinical Psychological Science*, 1(3), pp.239–252. doi:10.1177/2167702612471660.

Jayne's situation involved a particular kind of objective. She sought to remain professionally relevant in a field in which ageism is common. An interesting 2010 study out of Finland is worth noting in this regard, as it focused particularly on cosmetic patients older than age fifty-five.[5] Through interviews, the researchers explored the reasons older patients cited for seeking these interventions. The author found that many patients were like Jayne in that they did not seek to deny aging but rather to diminish physical signs of certain emotions associated with aging. Like Jayne, several of the patients spoke of goals such as looking content and self-confident, rather than angry, cynical, or tired. Patients referenced seeking changes that would combat social stereotypes of older people that cause them to be perceived as inactive, unhealthy, and irrelevant.

Most poignantly, some subjects in the Finnish study spoke of feeling unhappy because they no longer recognized their image in the mirror. They sought a cosmetic procedure simply to "become themselves" again. Also like Jayne, several of them considered the surgical procedure to be a means of recovering from a particularly stressful period in their life, such as a divorce or the death of a spouse. "I must erase those years from my face," one interviewee stated.

The above studies find that patients often report satisfaction regarding the particular aesthetic change they sought. This suggests that patients like Jayne can feel confident that the right procedures, for the right reasons, can be quite beneficial.

---

5 Kinnunen, Taina. (2010). *A Second Youth: Pursuing happiness and respectability through cosmetic surgery in Finland.* Sociology of Health and Illness, 32(2), pp.258–271. doi: 10.1111/j.1467-9566.2009.01215.x.

Change and Growth within the Context of Pain and Grief

Like some of the subjects in the study out of Finland, Jayne consulted a physician because she wanted to accomplish a kind of erasing of the effects of certain life events. For Jayne, the objective was grief-related. Though she had not experienced the death of a loved one, Jayne had experienced the sudden death of the way she viewed her husband, her marriage, and her closest friendship. That's a lot of erasing. It's a lot to ask of a surgeon. Fortunately, Jayne was psychologically sophisticated enough to realize she needed to heal from within to achieve the ultimate goals she had for the procedure.

Jayne and I worked together using short-term, goal-directed psychotherapy methods. Those methods stress the importance of adopting healthy thought, feeling, and behavior patterns. In this type of psychotherapy, the central objective is always accurate thinking. This does not mean denial of pain; it means we see our emotional and physical sources of pain within their proper contexts. We see the whole picture.

The Whole Picture

Like most of the tools utilized in goal-directed psychotherapy, seeing the whole picture is not a new or complicated idea. This is the way people have coped with disappointments for many years. "It's not the end of the world" and "Play the hand you're dealt" are two of the many idioms proving this technique has intuitive value and has therefore helped people cope with difficult challenges for centuries. This is yet another example of interpreting events in a way that achieves balanced thinking by giving voice to the sources of gratitude, instead of focusing primarily on losses.

We need this kind of accurate perspective-taking to succeed in choosing kindness and self-compassion over toughness and judgment.

Toughness often involves denial of the things we reject—an "eyes on the prize" attitude. Both toughness and self-compassion are goal-directed, but self-compassion leaves room for acknowledging the inevitable setbacks along the way.

An example will help clarify how the "tough" way of coping does not leave room for inevitable disappointments. Consider, for instance, the experience of a less-than-optimal cosmetic outcome. A tough-minded response to this is actually quite common. It exhibits itself in a stubborn insistence on achieving the precise cosmetic objective the patient initially envisioned. This approach would be more likely to lead a patient to repeatedly seek corrective procedures until the outcome that was originally sought was achieved. This resembles perfectionism in that it sets a goal that is unlikely to be met. The predictable consequence is that, like the perfectionist, the patient feels perpetually unsatisfied.

The "tough-minded" patient might attribute their unhappiness to the failure of the procedure. But the truth would be the client's unhappiness stems from their own narrow, rigid, and excessive demands.

The alternative is to employ a kinder, more self-compassionate, and more forgiving perspective. This way of being leaves room for imperfect surgical outcomes. Although this outlook might still lead to a corrective procedure, it is less likely to lead to the perfectionistic, endless series of procedures tough-mindedness often spawns. In this way, a more compassionate mindset improves a person's ability to see the whole picture and thus to embrace the possibility of an imperfect outcome.

Self-Compassion and Recovery

For Jayne, self-compassion played a central role in her process of recovering emotionally from the divorce. The kindness and gentleness Jayne began directing toward herself helped her embrace her whole reality. The tough and demanding part of herself tended to insist that specific wrinkles or frowns be eliminated. A kinder and more self-respecting way of entering the procedure involved her leaving room for the possibility that the surgical outcome might not be exactly what she had envisioned. If she were to accept that reality, she would acquire more control over her satisfaction with the results.

I wanted to help Jayne relax her standards for feeling satisfied with the procedure. Since there is always uncertainty in cosmetic outcomes, I suggested that she take the initiative by defining a successful cosmetic outcome in a way that accounts for the uncertainty. I told her a realistic cosmetic goal would lessen the distress potential of a less-than-perfect outcome.

Jayne looked at me as though I was insane. In fact, she replied, "I love you dearly, but are you insane? I gave that man a check for twenty-eight thousand dollars. Do you realize that? Twenty-eight thousand dollars. If I come out looking like Cruella de Vil, I'm not going to be happy."

"Okay, I get that, but what if we imagine an outcome that's a little closer to what your ideal goal is than that?" I replied.

She paused and sat back on the couch. She took a deep breath and sat with her thoughts. When she spoke, her tone had lost the comic edge. "There are realities at work here. I'm pushing seventy. That's my reality. And I need this procedure to help me to dial that clock back. Otherwise it's a waste of my time."

"I think it's fine to have those positive expectations. You've found a great surgeon. You've spent a lot of money. What I wonder is, do they have to hinge on a narrow definition of positive aesthetic change? Can you allow a segment of your expectations to not be linked to what the surgeon does? Instead, can you link that portion of your expectations to your own inner growth and change process? I think if you can do that, you take some control back. Now the success is partially defined by you, apart from the physical changes."

Jayne did work on defining success in this broader way. In session, we discussed the idea that the procedure will address the effects of time and gravity, but that her own mindset will be the key to her reacquiring a more youthful, resilient, and hopeful perspective. Ultimately, Jayne was happy with the cosmetic outcome. Despite her surgeon's impressive skills, her satisfaction was directly related to her decision to enter the procedure ready to move forward in her life.

Her experience provides a great example of the way cosmetic surgery patients benefit if they commit to a holistic process of change, rather than merely relying on the surgical event to bring about the changes. The unpredictability of cosmetic outcomes suggests hopefulness should be tempered by a realistic perspective. Besides, as I've noted, even successful outcomes can be undermined by overly critical mood states. So, every cosmetic patient benefits from focused inner growth work.

Inner Growth Work

"Inner growth work" refers to the work Jayne needed to do to begin the process of personal growth and change well before the procedure. Jayne embraced the inner work wholeheartedly. She knew she needed to begin to transform the harshly critical thoughts and feelings she had been nurturing. She spoke openly about those during the therapy, months before the cosmetic procedure.

Jayne used the same negative self-talk exercise Peter used, filling in a table like the one shown below. For Jayne, the condemning messages consistently focused on her ex-husband and her ex-friend. Sometimes they were also focused on other people. In one of the sessions, Jayne noted,

"The situation was that I woke up on my ex-friend's birthday. The negative thoughts were that people can't be trusted, and I was a fool for trusting her. And then I thought about Rosalie, a mutual friend. I figured she probably knew of the affair and never admitted she knew. That led to my thinking that members of my marketing team probably suspected and never said anything. All of this led me to picture myself moving far away, away from everyone, and just retiring. Then I recall thinking that I should just stay but find new friends because none of them can be trusted."

Situation	Negative Self-Talk	Positive Self-Talk
My friend's birthday.	People can't be trusted. I was a fool for trusting her.	Stop being cynical. People can be trusted.
	Members of my team betrayed me.	I know *I* wouldn't betray my friend, so not *everyone* is untrustworthy.
	I should move away.	The people who work under me would be crushed if I were to leave.
	I need new friends.	There are people who love and support me.

Jayne's positive column tended to address the negative column elements, so her exercise had three columns instead of four. That's fine. It's good for the client to alter the exercises in ways that fit best with their particular needs and preferences.

"This is a good example of how one negative thought can lead to another and another," I noted.

"Yes, they really do tend to do that. I get into those states and it feels like rolling down a steep hill."

"That's a common experience with that exercise. Can you tell me about the positive thoughts, Jayne, and also how you transitioned to them? Did you intentionally try to stop the negative thoughts by shifting to the positive, or did you run out of the negative thoughts?"

"I think they ran out," Jayne replied. "I remember saying to myself, 'Stop being cynical', so maybe I shifted myself. Anyway, the first positive thought was 'Stop it! People can be trusted.' And then I thought, 'I know *I* wouldn't betray my friend, so not *everyone* is untrustworthy.' And then I recall thinking about the people who work under me, and I thought they'd be crushed if I were to pick up and leave. I need to remember that there are people who love and support me. A lot of them."

One of the real signs of progress for Jayne was the lightening of her mood. Over time, working on these issues in therapy helped her let go of her cynicism and distrust of others. Many people would not have been as successful as Jayne in this regard. Her success was a powerful testament to her inner strength and will.

Over time, she began to use a combination of self-compassion, gratitude, and future-envisioning exercises, plus meditation in the morning and before bedtime. These meditations were selected for their capacity to help her reactivate the positive attitude she'd had most of her life. She began to transition away from thoughts of betrayal and resentment and toward thoughts that focused on hopefulness and identifying the people and experiences she intended to bring into her life in the future.

Jayne used three different types of meditations regularly. One type focused on subjects. These meditations present an idea expressed in a paragraph, then an affirmation and a mantra. Then the meditator sits quietly and allows those ideas to coexist with her mind. The meditation subjects Jayne used are the ones presented in this book, at the end of

Chapter 12. Jayne found that it was most helpful for her to search the meditations by topic and choose the one that felt most relevant on the given day.

The second type of meditation Jayne used was a traditional mindfulness meditation. This one did not ask her to focus on a thought or idea. Instead, the objective was simply to sit with herself. I asked her to use this meditation to practice simply being present with any thought or perception that entered her mind. The objective is to practice being aware and yet not reactive in the face of thoughts or impulses. This use of mindfulness meditation helped her to practice coexisting with her thoughts in a way that felt like it was from a safer distance.

I reminded Jayne that, during the mindfulness meditation, the goal is to achieve awareness without judgment, but that's a tall order, even for experienced meditators. I urged her to simply notice her thoughts and feelings as she meditated and to not punish herself if she were to notice herself judging her thoughts or anything else that popped into her head. This is a way to practice self-compassion, compassion toward others, and curiosity.

Jayne and I discussed the importance of self-compassion in her process of transformation. Her divorce was a horrific experience during which she was treated terribly. She had to commit to honoring the part of herself that, understandably, felt hurt and vengeful. This required her to be present with those parts of herself and to adopt a compassionate posture toward herself, like that which she would expect a supportive friend to exhibit.

Jayne and I also worked on honoring the uniqueness of her experience. This helped her begin to better understand how she acquired the messages she would say to herself, about herself. Despite her independence, she acknowledged that she's human and had been influenced by demands that society pushes us to adopt even though they're often not healthy. For example, she realized that one of the demands she placed on herself was that she never be betrayed. She felt weak and like a failure because her ex-husband and friend had betrayed her trust. She believed she had failed herself.

Jayne used the work we did together in her psychotherapy along with the meditations to begin to choose to view the betrayals differently. Instead of taking the blame, she concluded that it had never been her fault and that it had been unfair to blame herself. Instead, she chose to work on forgiving the part of herself that trusted her husband and friend.

Another way Jayne worked on treating herself with more compassion and respect involved her bedtime routine. She began saying a brief mantra, repeating it several times before going to sleep. It was a positive, brief statement like the ones provided with the meditations in this book. An example would be "I respect myself." Another would be "I feel myself evolving." Another that Jayne used was "I deserve to have pleasant dreams and thoughts." These helped her to stop ending and beginning each day by compulsively reactivating negative thoughts and feelings about her ex-husband and ex-friend.

Gratitude and Tonglen Meditation

There is one final type of meditation I gave Jayne that she found especially helpful. It is based on the Tonglen meditation technique. I encouraged Jayne to consider it a gratitude meditation. Tonglen meditations are not usually described as gratitude exercises, but they can certainly serve that function, and this is the way I typically use Tonglen meditations when I recommend them to my clients. Below you will find the formal instruction I provided Jayne for this meditation.

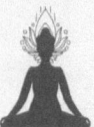

Exercise: Tonglen Meditation for Enhancing Feelings of Gratitude

Reminder: a guided version of this meditation is located at DrAlanGoodwin.com

1. Please sit in a comfortable, alert position and breathe in a way that relaxes you and helps you feel present with yourself.

2. Once you feel present, in your mind focus on a source of pain that causes you to struggle. For example, you might be coping with the sense that you have been betrayed, or you might be coping with a loss. When you choose one, please sit with the feelings that arise. Notice all physical feelings, thoughts, and emotions. Be a compassionate and curious observer of all of it. If you find yourself becoming consumed by any of them, try to gently bring your focus back to being a compassionate observer. Devote enough time to this part to be clear about the nature of your struggle.

3. Now, as you focus on your breathing, bring your focus back to your presence in the room. When you feel present, focus on a source of comfort you rely on to cope with the struggle. This could be the comfort of

your meditation practice, or of time spent with loved ones, or of a pleasant activity, or it could be as simple as the comfort of sleeping in your bed. Please focus on that source of comfort. Devote time to sitting with and honoring the gratitude you feel for having access to that source of comfort that helps you cope with your struggle.

4. Next, return your focus to your breathing. Once you feel present with your breath, focus back on the source of the struggle you identified earlier. Please think broadly about that struggle. For instance, the source of your struggle might have been betrayal, or loss, or physical pain. As you focus on the source of that pain, recognize that your pain is one that people have experienced all around the world for many, many years. In fact, there must be many, many thousands of other people in the world, right now, who are struggling with the same issue as you. As you focus on this fact, allow yourself to recognize that many of those people do not have access to an effective source of comfort, like the one that comforts you as you endure the struggle. As you continue to use your breathing to remain present, allow yourself to be aware of the struggle similar to your own that, for many people throughout the world is not yet diminished by sources of comfort.

5. Now, as you breathe, please imagine that with every inhale, you breathe in your awareness of the struggle that those people share with you. Pause briefly after

each inhale, noticing your compassion for them. Allow nice long exhales. And with every exhale, imagine that your exhale sends your wish that each of those people will find a source of comfort like the one you have found. Breathe as though your breath sends that wish out into the universe. Continue this generous, grateful, compassionate breathing as long as you'd like to.

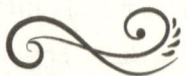

CHAPTER 5

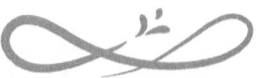

Beyond the Mirror: Other People's Reactions to Cosmetic Changes

Rocks are thrown only at fruit-bearing trees.

—*Japanese Proverb*

Cosmetic Change in the Age of the Fishbowl

"Hi! My favorite doctor in the world said you're fabulous and I should talk with you. So, let's talk." That was the way twenty-six-year-old Ayesha introduced herself to me. An actress, model, and social influencer, Ayesha was a dynamic person. She tended to present herself as optimistic, energetic, warm, attractive, engaging, and fearlessly fashion-forward. She wore cream-colored thigh-high boots and a conservative, color-matched dress and cashmere sweater to her first session. I remember it because I commented on her meticulous sense of style. Even in the first moments of the initial session, she replied with self-awareness, saying the comment helped her to feel seen and affirmed.

Ayesha always stood out. Throughout our work together, her clothing choices consistently struck an orchestrated balance between edgy and tasteful. She put a lot of thought into how she appeared. As a social influencer, the world she chose was a giant fishbowl. She was committed to making an impact in it. And she did. She had an abundance of friends, fans, and followers.

Soon after getting to know Ayesha, I realized her favorite physician was a psychologically sophisticated cosmetic surgeon who had referred patients to me in the past. The surgeon's reasons for referring Ayesha were clear within minutes of first talking with her. Ayesha was an attractive young woman who exhibited an alarming urgency to receive multiple cosmetic interventions.

Her doctor was concerned about the intensity of Ayesha's desires. Six weeks prior to our meeting, Ayesha had received two separate nonsurgical cosmetic services (fillers and Botox) from this doctor. Her doctor told her not to evaluate the results until at least six weeks after the procedures. Ayesha enthusiastically returned to the surgeon six weeks to the day after the procedures. Although she felt satisfied with the results, Ayesha now sought several more procedures. When her doctor hesitated and suggested she reconsider, Ayesha stated her mind was made up.

Ayesha and her surgeon were at a stalemate on the subject of her undergoing additional procedures so soon after the prior ones. The surgeon later informed me that his advice to Ayesha to delay more procedures did not involve medical concerns; he was only concerned about her psychological health. When Ayesha refused to accept the surgeon's advice to delay more cosmetic work, he offered her a deal: if Ayesha would meet twice with a psychologist to discuss her cosmetic procedure plans, the surgeon would meet with her again to discuss her objectives. Ayesha agreed to that deal.

It usually doesn't bode well when a client comes to you because someone told them to. Usually, people who benefit from psychotherapy choose it themselves. Despite this, it turned out Ayesha was wonderfully open and engaged in her psychotherapy with me. We met many more times than the required two sessions. In our initial session, she explained she had already begun searching for a psychologist when her surgeon urged her to contact me.

Ayesha's presentation had become very important to her. That was by design: her physical identity was central to her business model. As a young and attractive transgender woman, she intended to create a public image that she could monetize. Popularly defined beauty, she decided, was an essential element of her value. She considered her positive outlook on life to be another tool of influence. She was in that fishbowl and she was decked out in sequin and diamonds.

Social Media and the Pressure to Change

People who are successful social media influencers constantly monitor their online presence. The ones who succeed are smart, and Ayesha was no exception. Her success, she explained, required an intense focus on establishing and maintaining her brand, which she also labeled her "public vibe."

"It's not just about looking hot," she explained. "That's always a part of it. But it's also about the vibe. It's about showing people how to have fun, enjoy life."

"So, help me understand, do you film every day?"

"Every day," Ayesha replied, in a tone that indicated it was a burdensome task.

"From your tone, I gather there are days when you just don't want to be filmed?"

"Oh, there are days when I don't even want to be seen—by anyone. But you know, the show must go on." As Ayesha continued, her tone lightened. "The camera is always on. Not really, but it feels like that. I really don't mind it. I rarely have an entire day when I don't film." She stopped and seemed to be reconsidering her comments. "Look, I'm not gonna lie to you. It's an issue, at times. I mean, it's a lot. Actually, one reason for the cosmetic work is it can save me time preparing prior to filming. Covering up the issues, I mean."

"I'm not sure what you mean by that, Ayesha. Do you feel comfortable telling me what some of the issues are that you're referring to?"

"Oh honey, let's just say what you see when you look at me is not what the mirror sees when I brush my teeth in the morning. This," she said, framing her face with her hands, "is a lot of work. Work and maintenance, baby. Work and maintenance. There are dozens and dozens of bits and pieces. A dark spot here, contouring there, raising this, lowering that, highlighting this, hiding that. There are a lot of minor details that need to be addressed. When taken together, well, it's a lot."

"Are you saying the cosmetic procedures save you time because your makeup doesn't have to cover up so many of the cosmetic issues you're alluding to?" I asked.

"Yes. Definitely. Effective procedures have saved me hours, and I've saved hundreds of dollars every few months on makeup I no longer need to buy. For instance, I had my nose corrected a while ago. That eliminated the need for certain contouring. Since then, peels, laser treatments, and injections have blurred pores and reduced sun damage issues that I had previously covered every day. I also had acne scarring. I don't have to cover up the way I used to."

"On the subject of covering up, I'm impressed by how expertly you learned to do these things. How did you learn so much about shadowing and other methods of using makeup?"

"I've been studying it for years. YouTube, mainly," she said.

"I see. Do you feel comfortable telling me more about the injections you've sought? I'm curious to know what function they served."

"Sure. For me, injections are about correcting proportionality. They helped correct the shape of my face. But injections are dicey. You really need to be careful. For instance, I'll get my lips done again, but only by the same doctor. I won't become one of those girls who ruin themselves by trying to save a few dollars on lip work. You just can't do that. Not with lips. I've only gone to places where doctors do the work on me."

"As you describe these plans," I said, "I'm struck by how precise you are. Everything seems to be well-researched. Have you regretted any of the procedures?"

"Actually, I haven't regretted any, yet." She had a tendency to stand up during our sessions and stroll around the room. She said it helped her think. I jokingly told her once that I thought she stood so I could see her shoes, which were consistently noteworthy. We often eased into sessions by beginning with her description of any great shoe-finds during the past week. On this day, she informed me she wore high-heeled slingback sandals. When I observed they appeared to be yellow snakeskin, she clarified that the color was actually "lemonade constrictor" and that they were, in fact, completely vegan and humanely and sustainably produced, with a portion of the proceeds donated to charities promoting animal welfare. Boa-cruelty-free.

For some people, standing up and walking during the session would be a symptom of avoidance. Not with Ayesha. In this instance, she stood as she discussed her approach to undergoing cosmetic services. "I'm very careful," she continued. "Like I said, I've seen some disastrous cosmetic work. So, I try to be strategic. I choose the procedures very carefully, and I choose the doctors even more carefully. I know what I want, and I've found people who can give it to me."

"Ayesha, it's important to me that my clients trust me to be transparent and direct. I look at you and I see a woman the world considers to be beautiful. So it seems to me you've done a very good job so far. I wonder, though, if you might one day lose perspective. Your physical image is such a central aspect of your public identity. Isn't it hard to maintain your perspective with all the comments you must hear and read? Does your own voice get crowded out sometimes?"

She walked swiftly to her seat on the sofa. She sat and said, with conviction, "It's hard. I try to listen. But everyone, EV-REE-ONE, has an opinion. And they all want to tell you it. I listen to the doctors but, to be honest, between my followers and the haters, I hear the brutal truth. And they're the ones who count."

"They're the ones who count?" I repeated.

Ayesha rolled her eyes and smiled. "Okay, okay, I count too. Are you happier now?" She laughed. "Just keeping it real, honey. At the end of the day, this is a business, and they're paying my bills. I'm a big girl and I chose this business, you know? I chose this. And I just think, if I'm gonna do it, I need to do it. Go big or go home."

"I understand. You're saying your appearance is central to your business model, and these procedures have been a necessary aspect of that."

"Exactly," Ayesha said.

"And you said a minute ago that sometimes it's hard to hear your own voice, above the followers and haters. Does that mean you worry you might lose perspective sometime? That you might overdo it with the cosmetic work?"

"I know there's a risk. I'm aware." She sounded curt, so I suspected she might have felt irritated by my pressing the issue.

"Does it bother you that I asked again whether you worry about the risk of overdoing the procedures?"

"Well, I guess so. But no. No. I want you to ask me what you think I need to be asked. I mean, look, I've seen girls go overboard, okay? I've seen it. And I've seen it in the boys, too, by the way. We've all seen them. The eyes, the nose, the hips, the cheekbones, the ass...like I said, honey, some fools ruin themselves. But I really think my followers, the sane ones, tell me what I need to hear. I do trust them. Good doctors are important but, to be honest, I look for a doctor who can do what I want, not one who wants to tell me what they think I should want. I know what I want. I know my brand better than any doctor does."

"I believe you," I said. "You seem so laser-focused on your career. Can we shift our focus just a bit? I'm curious to know more about your resilience. I can't help but wonder how you cope with the haters, the less sane followers. Can you talk a little about that?"

"I read their comments once, and then I move on," Ayesha said.

"Really? You can do that? You don't think about the comments after reading them?"

"Clocked!" Ayesha said. She had a big laugh; she really exploded in laughter, here. Shaking her head, she continued, "I need to be real with you. So, I do think about them, okay? I do. I stay up nights, sometimes, thinking about those fools. And they definitely make me check myself in the mirror sometimes. Like I said, it's hard."

"I would think it'd be really hard to read the hateful content," I said.

As Ayesha responded, she flicked a speck off her slacks, speaking with the matter-of-fact tone again. "It's not fun, but I'm used to it now." During our work together, Ayesha often shifted to that matter-of-fact tone. For her, it was a temporary defense. She'd usually come back around pretty quickly to being real again with me. She'd usually do that without my even having to draw her attention to it. This is one of the ways she was very self-aware.

Ayesha's matter-of-factness served the same function that humor serves in serious situations. It was a way to reduce tension. In our sessions, she'd use it to buy time. It made sense that she would need that time to remind herself that the therapy room was a safe place for her to be herself. In her world, she was accustomed to avoiding any mention of negative feelings.

Clients often worry about the vibe in the therapy room. They ask me how I can hear so much negativity all day long. They worry about over-burdening me. In response, I usually tell them that I don't think of our pain as destructive. I explain that, if we view the struggles of life as normal aspects of our humanity, we are better able to embrace them. In this way, we can see the opportunities for growth that lie within our difficulties.

Maintaining Independence within the Context of Social Adoration

The work with Ayesha needed to focus on helping her preserve her sense of independence. The problem wasn't as simple, though, as Ayesha suffering from an addiction to being adored. Some social media influencers do seem to suffer from that. At this point in our work together, I wasn't convinced Ayesha had that problem. The way she described it, she viewed the adoration as a necessary aspect of her business model. I suspected it wasn't that simple, but I was hopeful to learn more about this as our work unfolded.

Like so many people, and especially women, Ayesha's self-image was influenced by an oppressive sea of social pressures that dictated how her face and body should look.

The impact of those messages was intensified by her ubiquitous presence on social media platforms. To add to the problem, she felt "all in," as she often said, explaining defiantly that "I've invested too much time and effort in this career to just bail on it now. That is not going to happen. So, I need to maintain myself."

As a trans woman, there was the added social pressure that arose out of her role as a mentor for trans women and other marginalized people. She valued her independence, but she also embraced her beauty. Particularly for women, it can be difficult to maintain both of those values because beauty is so often dictated by society's rigid standards. And those demands regarding her appearance were communicated frequently and explicitly to her because of her social media presence.

I felt like I needed to reassure her. I explained, "Ayesha, it's important that you know that I really don't have an agenda to convince you to abandon your social media identity. And I also don't think it's my job to talk you into or out of a cosmetic procedure. In fact, I think it would be disrespectful if I were to try to do that. I know that you know what you want, and I know you've done your research. My job is to help you take good care of yourself. Mainly, that's accomplished by my collaborating with you to help you look within. Your answers will come from you, not from me."

Ayesha had only experienced brief psychotherapy prior to our work. She reported her prior experience had been pleasant, but not impactful. Initially, I believed there were several issues to address in psychotherapy with her. First, there was the adoration issue. We needed to continue to examine her relationship with her followers' adoration. Second, she needed to examine the very rigid definition she had adopted of beauty. And third, Ayesha needed to gain a better understanding of how she had learned to devalue the parts of herself that were not tied to being adored—both physically and emotionally. In other words, away from her social media platform, she needed to be more intentional about seeing herself as a whole person, rather than merely as a tool for other people's entertainment and adoration. We discussed these goals, and Ayesha felt comfortable with the plan to pursue them.

One of the exercises Ayesha found very helpful was the "My Change Process" journaling exercise provided at the end of Chapter 3. That journaling exercise gave her the chance to get clearer about the ways being an influencer had altered how she treated herself. She did not want to give up her celebrity status, but she did decide to work on enhancing her ability to feel genuine self-compassion and self-acceptance. One of the changes she made in this regard was that she chose to detach more often from social media.

Even more than the journaling work, Ayesha benefited from mindfulness and meditation. At the end of this chapter, I've provided the loving kindness meditation she found most useful. Once she became exposed to the power of meditation, Ayesha began meditating daily. The meditations she used are scattered throughout this book. Ayesha indicated that she found the journaling and meditation work to be transformational. She once said she felt that "meditation is like holding a mirror up to my mind."

Ayesha found the compassionate focus of the loving kindness meditation to be especially empowering. It clarified her view of other people. "I feel like I see the struggle in people more clearly, now. It jumps out at me when I observe them," she once said. Meditation helped her humanize her friends, the people who aren't her friends, and herself. The recognition of their shared struggle is the essence of compassion and it is the fuel of resilience. This explains her sense of empowerment.

Resilience: Coping with the Followers and the Haters

Ultimately, Ayesha developed much more resilience. She came to see herself differently in some important ways. Being attractive was still part of her brand, but she developed much more clarity about where the boundary stood between other people's adoration of her and her own self-esteem. She spent a fair amount of time using meditations and mantras that reinforced her sense of self-acceptance and respect. In this way, Ayesha became even more self-assured and resilient.

We frequently discussed resilience in the process of helping her normalize the struggles and barriers life sent her way. We explored the role resilience can play in life. Resilient people confront the same obstacles, but they respond to them assertively.

Ayesha entered therapy as a smart, successful businesswoman. Still, she tended to be overly reactive to the feedback she received on social media. She acquired more resilience when she decided to listen more to her own intuition and less to the feedback from her followers. She also decided to set new limits on how much of herself she gave to them. So, for instance, she decided to cancel plans to undergo one of the cosmetic treatments she had planned.

A more difficult change occurred in the frequency of Ayesha's online presence. Gradually, Ayesha learned to trust that she could take some days off. Previously, she had felt driven to post content almost continuously. Her prolific presence was one of the reasons she grew her online brand so effectively. But she often felt exhausted. The exhaustion convinced her to listen more carefully to her body and mind, and helped her to focus more on nurturing the joy within herself.

Ayesha reported that the meditation work was primarily responsible for her decision to take more time off. "I began the meditation practice with very brief meditations," she explained. "Like two minutes here and there. And I used positive mantras. The more I did them, the more I noticed that I felt more calm. So, I started doing them for four minutes and then eight minutes and so on. I think the mindfulness meditations helped me the most when I was posting really often. Meditation helped me feel how different I felt when I was so busy posting. I just feel so much more present now. Without meditation, I don't think I would have noticed what it felt like to really be present. I still post a lot, but I try to be aware of being present. I feel much more authentic now."

"Do you find the meditation practice has impacted how you feel about yourself?" I asked.

"I definitely do feel differently about myself. It sounds corny, but I really do feel the self-compassion. I appreciate myself more. I feel kinder, including to myself."

Coping with Loss of Privacy and Judgmental Reactions

Some patients worry that others will know they underwent a cosmetic procedure. This is especially true of public figures. Celebrities, for example, often feel pressured to be both beautiful and ageless. As a result, the appearance of even a successful procedure is often not desirable. When these concerns arise, they can undermine surgical outcomes by altering the patient's health-related behaviors.

Women often confront a particular set of concerns related to the reactions of others. In some communities, any elective procedure is considered inappropriate. Women are especially likely to be discouraged from choosing cosmetic work. It isn't unusual for women to report feeling shamed by others because they were believed to have indulged themselves with a cosmetic procedure.

This source of stress tends to be particularly intense in women who are mothers, regardless of the age of their children. Mothers are socialized in many cultures to always place the needs of others ahead of their own needs. Women who are mothers often discuss their concern that others will judge them for spending so much money on themselves, rather than on their children. Mothers often worry they will be labelled selfish, unstable, vain, or a combination of these. This anxiety makes choosing an expensive cosmetic service particularly difficult for them. A routine post-op trip to a salon, grocery store, or school parent night can turn into a grueling emotional experience if the patient perceives gossip about them or receives direct questions about their procedure.

The Unique Challenges for Male Patients

The experience of the male cosmetic surgery patient can also be fraught with complex challenges. Although men are encouraged to maintain good hygiene, they are not encouraged to be openly concerned about their personal attractiveness. In the past couple of decades gender roles have certainly become more relaxed, particularly in large cities. Still, it's common for male patients to worry that cosmetic alterations will be perceived as feminine. My clinical experience has been that men still usually feel discouraged from disclosing their cosmetic enhancements to other people.

A slightly different issue arises when the cosmetic improvement a man seeks involves appearing more muscular. On the one hand, a male patient may feel admired due to his newly muscular physique, which can be partially achieved, for instance, after undergoing a successful 4D VASER liposuction procedure with fat transfer. Still, that man will often feel judged as someone who has cut corners and not "earned" other people's admiration if others learn his impressive build was kick-started by a surgical procedure. The reality is, 4D VASER liposuction provides only a kick-start. The patient needs to adopt an appropriate muscle-building exercise and diet regimen if he is going to achieve optimal muscular development. But haters will be haters, so there will always be people who wrongly assume a muscular man who had this procedure didn't have to work hard to achieve it.

So, male cosmetic patients may feel stigmatized for a variety of reasons. In psychotherapy, they struggle with these judgments. Men often discuss their concern that they will be criticized as insecure, weak, and less "manly" if they seek a cosmetic improvement. Understandably, those who fear the negative stigma of being a cosmetic surgery patient are much more likely to feel protective of their medical privacy. In my experience, in Los Angeles, physicians who specialize in cosmetic procedures for men have an acute appreciation for these issues.

Permafrost and Privacy

Effective psychotherapy encourages the patient to accept their reality. Ideally, medical privacy protections ensure that other people will only learn about a patient's cosmetic procedure if the patient tells them about it. In the real world, this is unfortunately not always the case. Particularly when the patient is a celebrity, the public sometimes learns of the procedure. Psychotherapy clients who are public figures often need to prepare for this possibility, and they frequently fear the loss of medical privacy. As the following client experience demonstrates, the concern can be intensified by the nature of the patient's profession.

Gwen, a fifty-two-year-old, high-powered litigation attorney, was born and raised in Muncie, Indiana. She and her four siblings, all younger than Gwen, were raised by their two parents in a small two-bedroom home. Gwen earned her law degree from the University of Notre Dame and immediately relocated to Los Angeles. When Gwen sought my help, she was not yet a public figure. She would later acquire notoriety because of her central role in a case involving a public figure.

Gwen came to me to explore the risks and benefits of aesthetic work. She planned to have upper and lower blepharoplasty procedures because she believed her eyes caused her to look tired and older. She was of the opinion that these procedures sometimes produced an outcome that caused the patient's face to appear unnatural, and she remained unsure whether to go through with the procedure.

Gwen was concerned that if her planned procedures were to fail, she could lose credibility as an attorney. "I've seen men and women come back after being away for some months," she explained, "and it's obvious they had work done." As Gwen spoke, she manipulated a fountain pen she held, rolling, flipping, and twirling it with only the fingers of her right hand. She never looked at the pen. She seemed to use it as a concentration tool, the way some people use knitting. "The surgical results I've seen are much worse than the permafrost Botox face. These people do have that, but they also have the deer-in-the-headlights sort of exaggerated stare, or the stationary and raised eyebrows, or the sort of triangulation-face some people acquire due to bad use of fillers. It's disconcerting because, as a patient, you have to wonder where the butchers are who are performing those procedures. I don't think I've run into a physician who would do that kind of work, but how can I know for sure, until the deed has been done?"

"Gwen, you describe those changes in clever ways that are funny, but I hear the very serious concerns you have."

This comment seemed to calm Gwen. She set her pen on the end table next to her, leaving her hand on the table, her index finger resting on the pen. There had been a presentational quality to her description of poorly executed cosmetic surgeries. I wanted to help her ease down into the sofa and sit a bit more authentically with her fears. This also gave me a chance to assess the degree to which, at this point, Gwen was available to receive my help. I was happy to see she was quite open and receptive. Gwen's tone immediately lost most of the affectedness as she replied, "Those kinds of changes make a person look worse than tired." After a brief pause, she pronounced, "I would never want to look the way those people look," as she crossed her legs and leaned back into the sofa.

"That's really helpful to me. I've worked with a lot of patients considering a cosmetic procedure, and it's pretty common for people to want to look revitalized, but not surgically corrected. People often stress that they don't want to dramatically alter their appearance. That's what I think I hear you saying. Does that describe how you feel?"

"It does," she said. "I think I can help you understand my motives a little better. I'm a litigator. I know you're an attorney, but I tell you I'm a litigator to tell you that I engage in negotiations all day, every day. Even when we're just talking, it's part of the negotiation process. Every lawsuit is really just protracted negotiation. You know, negotiations are often described as a dance, but any good attorney knows that's a ridiculous analogy. They're more like a judo match. The attorneys continually engage in moves and countermoves. It's all about leverage, balance, and dominance. Litigation attorneys are fighters, always looking for ways to aggress against their opposing counsel. Older male attorneys do this all the time. And they often fight dirty. A surprising number of them are real pricks. You'd be surprised."

In my role as a psychologist, I try to avoid using the brief experiences I had as an active attorney. In this case, however, I decided to break my rule because it gave me an opportunity to align with Gwen, which was important at this stage in our clinical work. So I interjected, "Just so you know, actually, I wouldn't be surprised at how unnecessarily obnoxious litigators can be. I saw it when I was a young litigator. I remember it happening even in the elevator, on the way to or from a hearing."

"Oh sure. The elevator is a great spot for a snide remark. Okay, so you get it," Gwen replied.

"Still, please share the details. I had much less experience than you. And, as a young man, I'm sure my experiences were very different from yours. I believe your description of your experience, and I'm sorry you've had to deal with that."

"Thank you. I'm sorry too," Gwen said. "You know, sometimes they'd make indirect reference to my gender. Years ago, they'd try to use my age, plus my gender, against me. A casual observer might hear the comments as innocent remarks, even compliments, but I always know exactly what the jerk-of-the-day is doing. And he knows what he's doing, too. It's all part of the fight. All part of the process of trying to use my youth and gender against me, to remind me he was bigger and stronger. Lawyers like those guys will look for any personal characteristic to try to gain an advantage over their opposing counsel."

"Your awareness of those behaviors will be very helpful to our work together. I'm glad you were able to trust me enough to tell me about those experiences. You sound really observant and resilient."

"Thank you," Gwen replied. "It's nice to feel seen."

The Sensei Within

Gwen was smart and introspective. I wasn't surprised to find that she engaged actively in her psychotherapy. We focused on strengthening her resilience. In particular, in preparation for her surgical procedure, our work focused on preserving her competitive edge yet maintaining a healthy detachment from other people's behaviors and judgments.

At this point, it's important to discuss Gwen's martial arts training. Years prior to our meeting, she earned a black belt in judo. She was an active judoka at the time of our meetings. Gwen had been training for many years with a particular judo sensei, or instructor. She viewed her sensei as a mentor not only in terms of judo technique, but also in terms of her spiritual life.

I commented once, "Gwen, when you talk about your judo training, I hear such reverence from you toward your sensei, and toward the practice in general."

"It's true," she said. "On your website, you describe the role mindfulness plays in the work you do with clients. That was one of the reasons I contacted you. Mindfulness has played a central role in my judo training. The role of the mind, and the objective of finding inner peace, are both issues I've been examining for over twenty years. I began the practice when I started training with my sensei. It's been transformational. I know who I am. I know what I value."

"Anyone who looks at you can see that you appear very self-assured. I'm sure part of that is related to the practice of law, because looking that way is functional. But I wonder about your internal experience, your sense of self. Another way of saying this is your level of self-respect. At a deep level, has that been part of your spiritual practice?"

"Well, that's not a simple subject. On the one hand, we are definitely not trained to be timid or to doubt ourselves, and yet, the philosophy of judo is rooted in respect and compliance. We comply with the aggressor's actions. This is what I was referring to when I said we use their aggression against them."

"Gwen, that is so interesting, because meditation is really a way to practice acceptance and not resisting. I mean, in a sense, our thoughts are aggressing against us, sometimes. In meditation, we practice coexisting with them because if we resist them, their power over us grows. So, meditation is also about complying, except in meditation, we comply with our own thoughts to allow them to flow out of us. The power of meditation is that it helps us to practice not resisting. This helps us to tolerate the things we dislike."

Gwen sat back in the armchair. She seemed to be deep in thought. "I always think of meditation as a way to chill. My sensei teaches us to use our breath to re-center ourselves. I never really drew the connection to my thinking. That's different but consistent with what my sensei teaches."

"So, you covered the compliance piece just now. What about the self-respect piece? How have you been taught to view yourself?"

"Humility is important. You earn respect by your behavior. But you're asking something different. You're asking about my inner sense of self. If I'm honest, the answer is I can play the part. I can claim to possess a strong sense of self-respect. But I know you're not asking about appearances." Gwen sat and thought for a couple of minutes as she slowly nudged the pen with her index finger, forward a bit, then back a bit. "It's tough," she said. "I don't think I have the authentic self-confidence down yet."

"Does that play a role in the decision about whether to undergo the procedure?" I asked.

"It does. For sure." She picked up the pen and pointed it toward me for emphasis as she spoke, each thought a proclamation. "I think that's why I'm here. This procedure should not be about rejecting who I am. I'm a fifty-two-year-old grown-ass woman. I'm strong and healthy. I want to embrace that. I *need* to embrace that. I need to embrace my age and experience and the changes in my body. And yet," she said, setting the pen down, her tone turning to resignation, "I want to remain relevant. My face is part of my armor. It's one of the weapons I rely on. I need to maintain it."

"I can understand the conflicting feelings within you. But it sounds like you feel convinced the procedure is the right thing for you to do."

"I think it is. But I feel defeated, somehow. I can't explain it. Even before I've done it, before I've seen any result, I feel defeated."

"Do you notice how much you use combat imagery, Gwen?"

"I feel like a fighter. I fight all day long as a litigator."

"And you said you rely on your face. It's one of your weapons, you said."

"Yes," Gwen replied, "I did. It is. I've never discussed that with my sensei. I think he'd feel disappointed. Spiritually, I embrace human vulnerabilities like aging. Professionally, I view vulnerabilities in others as issues to use in my favor or, when in myself, as issues to eliminate. This is why I'm considering the procedure. My face needs to be effective."

"So, there is some conflict between the spiritual values and the professional ones?"

"My sensei would definitely say there is." Gwen laughed. "That's why I haven't told him these things."

"And your face is like a samurai sword that needs sharpening from time to time?"

"You're not making it easier," Gwen said, laughing.

"I really don't mean to imply you shouldn't use your face as a weapon, or that you shouldn't maintain it. I'm just wanting to shine a light on the analogy."

"Well, I don't feel wonderful about it. But I need to be competitive in my field."

"Absolutely," I said. "What's interesting to me is that you described your work as involving modern-age forms of battle. Within that context, you compared the role your face plays to that of a sword, rather than, say, a shield."

Gwen smiled and sat back in the armchair, her index finger again finding the pen to slowly tap and rest on. "Okaaaay," she said, still smiling and nodding slowly as she thought more about the implications of seeing her face as an offensive weapon rather than as a defensive, protective one. She remained silent for a couple more minutes, continuing to nod, and then looked back at me and quietly said, "Touché. Touché."

Gwen's tone suggested she was enjoying our dialogue in the way a practitioner responds to a training partner. Her use of the word "touché" was helpful to me. It alerted me that my words might have sounded competitive. I don't want a client to feel as though they need to thrust and parry when they're speaking with me, so I addressed that.

"Isn't 'touché' something that's said after an effective strike? Did my comment about your face being a sword and not a shield feel aggressive or critical?" I asked.

"I suppose so, in a sense. I know you meant well. I don't feel injured by it. I think it was helpful. A helpful act of aggression," she concluded, laughing. After a pause she continued, "You know, I was drawn to judo because it's a practice that essentially relies on use of the opponent's momentum. As a trained judoka, I can throw a person who's twice my size even though I couldn't lift that person. I think that's what you were doing with me. You were using my momentum. That's why I'm smiling. That's what my saying 'touché' was about."

We smiled and sat in the silence. Then Gwen said, "So, my face as a shield. I need to sit with that. I need to think over what that means in terms of my surgery plans. Shields can have dents and scratches. They still protect."

"In fact, shields are made to be scratched and dented, right? Unless they're intended to be decorative."

"Yes. The dilemma lies in the fact that I like my shield to be decorative when I want it to be, but I also want it to be ready to provide protection when I need that."

"It seems like one of the things it might be helpful for us to explore together is the nature of your reliance on your face as a weapon. In other words, can you direct your mindfulness practice toward noticing how you use your face in various settings and with various people, and for what purposes?"

"I can," Gwen replied. "I think I need to do that. I need to wrestle with this dilemma a bit more, I think."

"Great," I said. 'see you next week."

One Hell of a Mimosa

We are all complex. Gwen's particular history made the complexity of our work together particularly compelling—for both of us. I was impressed with the way this martial arts expert and skilled litigation attorney so openly and courageously engaged in the process. She didn't hold up a mirror to herself; she held up an electron microscope. With precision and curiosity, she explored her personality, her life goals, her values, and the ways she thought of and treated herself. And she examined the ways these had continually been influenced by the intersectionality among her profession, her personal life, and her identity as a judo practitioner.

In Gwen's therapy, she had to confront the very real possibility that she might encounter public criticism after altering her appearance. We devoted a fair amount of time to examining how such reactions might wound her. Our process ultimately helped her reach her goal of feeling more empowered and resilient. During one of our sessions, she presented me with a conclusion that was a revelation of sorts to her.

"I was thinking this past Sunday about the subject of our work," she began. "I'd gone to a nice Italian brunch spot in Hermosa Beach. I was enjoying the sun and a mimosa and was just reflecting. I thought, you know, I encounter a lot of angry people. This is my reality, as an attorney. There's always unnecessary fighting. And I'm obliged to be ready to fight. If some asshole opposing counsel is a fighter, I need to fight."

"Sometimes you feel duty-bound to fight, even if it seems unnecessary?" I asked.

"Even if unnecessary," Gwen affirmed, in a resigned tone. Then she relaxed back deeper into the sofa, glancing at the Japanese gong I have in my office. I'd used it to facilitate meditations with her. She held her gaze on the gong for a minute or so, a long time. Then she calmly continued, "I thought about what you said about not personalizing the struggles of other people. It occurred to me, for years, my fights have been propelled by my decision to take other people's struggles personally. They were insulting *me*. They were trying to beat *me*. Now, to be honest, those men who tried to dominate me were struggling. I knew that. I always knew that. But I still resented their behavior toward me."

"So, you knew they were unhealthy, and you knew their unhealthiness explained their aggression against you, and yet their behavior felt personal."

"Yes," she replied, "it often did. And that was the epiphany on Sunday. I suddenly arrived at the recognition that my fighting was always related to my feeling that "I don't deserve that kind of treatment." I resented their behavior. I personally resented it. So, as I sat with the mimosa, feeling the sea breeze, and hearing birds chirping and the kids playing on the beach, I suddenly thought, 'What the fuck are you talking about? Of course you don't deserve it. It isn't even about you!' Then I thought, 'Why don't you get that?!' And then I think I got it in a way I never have before. I realized they were just being the assholes they were. I thought about what we discussed about allowing them to have their limitations. I thought of allowing them to be the assholes they are. It's been empowering. It's helped me to detach more thoroughly from their shit. Because—why stay attached to it?"

"That's right," I replied.

"I didn't cause it," Gwen continued.

"Nope, you sure didn't."

"And I don't deserve it."

"Nope, you sure don't," I said.

"And I can't stop it."

"That's for sure."

"So why should I be so invested in making them treat me well?" Gwen said. "So, moving forward, I feel much more prepared to see it, but not experience it as personal."

"That's awesome," I said. "It's really exciting to hear this." Then, after a pause, I added, "That place makes a hell of a mimosa!" We laughed.

Gwen decided to go through with the procedure. In the months that followed, she adopted a daily meditation practice. She reported she would do a guided fifteen-minute loving kindness meditation three to five days each week. Two to three days each week, Gwen did a guided ten-minute Tonglen meditation.

Gwen's psychotherapy continued to focus on helping her adopt new ways of reacting to the world. We used the Buddhist notion of treating other people who behave with unkindness as our "teachers." When other people behaved in these ways, Gwen was to focus on the struggle under-lying their behavior. In other words, she would interpret their behavior through a compassionate lens, rather than through a lens that was defen-sive and focused on self-protection.

The work Gwen was doing between sessions was really quite difficult. As Gwen said, tongue-in-cheek and sword-in-hand, when I first proposed it, "So, what you're telling me is you'd like me to look for opportunities to behave like a doormat."

"No. It's all about perspective," I replied. "Let me explain. The point of the exercise is to be aware of being stepped on while practicing not *feel-ing* stepped on. I know that sounds strange. It's about not taking things people do to us overly personally. Nobody enjoys being stepped on, but since other people's limitations will cause them to step on us sometimes, it's best for us to have tools that enable us to accept that and not take it so personally when it happens."

Gwen then said, "The truth is, I'm giving you a hard time even though I agree with you. You're essentially talking about judo—finding a way to use the aggressor's momentum against them."

"That's interesting. To be honest, I like borrowing only a part of that idea. Yes, like in judo, we are talking about using the other person's momentum. But for our purposes, it's not about using their momentum against them. Their momentum is exhibited in the limitations that cause them to struggle and therefore step on us. The idea is, if we accept that, in the way the judoka accepts the opponent's physical momentum, we, like the judoka, can use that information to determine the best way to respond. Are we in alignment, so far?"

"Yes," Gwen replied, "so far so good."

"Great. The only place where we diverge is I'm not suggesting that you use their momentum against them. I'm suggesting you use their momentum to reveal their struggle, helping you to respond with compassion rather than aggression."

Gwen smiled and said, "I think Sensei would approve."

Gwen and I discussed these questions at some length during the months that followed. The judo analogy entered into our discussions often. The type of judo Gwen studied fit very well with the mindfulness practices we used in her therapy. Over time, she improved her ability to resist personalizing other people's hostile behavior. This helped her feel less vulnerable as she prepared for and recovered from the procedure.

Compassion and the Unkindness of Strangers

This chapter focused on the difficult process of coping with the unsupportive forces we sometimes encounter. It's important to remember that the work with Gwen and Ayesha was for their benefit, not for the benefit of the people who might have behaved unkindly toward either of them. In preparing for their cosmetic services, they both practiced developing less sensitivity to other people's behavior.

That said, a primary focus in this chapter was on integrating compassion into our reactions to the unfriendly forces. The work was for Gwen and Ayesha, but there was plenty of room for compassion directed at the struggling and unsupportive people in their respective lives.

Ultimately, compassion was the reason both Ayesha and Gwen developed the ability to undergo their respective cosmetic interventions with much less fear surrounding the outcomes. They learned to detach more from other people's judgments and to listen to their own authentic voices. Fortunately for them, they had strong, clear voices. In the next chapter, we will explore some of the challenges people face when their inner voice is less friendly and supportive.

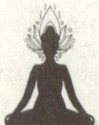

Exercise: Pure Mindfulness Meditation

The following is a pure form of mindfulness meditation. The practice tips provided for the Breath-focused Mindfulness Meditation at the end of Chapter 1 are appropriate for this meditation, as well. This more pure form of mindfulness meditation tends to be more difficult than a meditation that has a focal point, like counting your breaths. This meditation has no focus. Instead of attaching a number to your breaths, in this meditation you simply breathe and practice doing nothing else. Choose whichever type you want, or practice doing both. And remember, they are both difficult and you can begin with a meditation that is only one minute long.

Reminder: a guided version of this meditation is located at DrAlanGoodwin.com

Instructions for the meditation:

1. Find a quiet, private place.

2. Assume a comfortable, relaxed, alert position; upright, but not stiff.

3. Breathe. Stop. Be. Just take slow, deep breaths in and out.

4. Close your eyes or leave them open but resting on an object.

5. Notice whatever your five senses reveal to you. Take your time.

6. Exhale a bit longer than you inhale. Remain focused on your breathing. If your mind wanders to thoughts, notice that, allow it, then gently remind yourself to focus on your breath.

7. Try to let just breathing be enough. Allow thoughts to float into and out of your mind. If you engage a thought or two, notice that, and gently return your focus to your breath. Exhale a bit longer than you inhale.

8. When you feel ready to end the meditation, devote a few breaths to gratitude. Inhale feelings of gratitude. As you exhale, say a mantra or two silently or quietly, such as: *I am learning*, or *I am growing*, or *I feel blessed*.

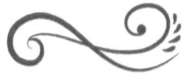

CHAPTER 6

The Enemy Within: Managing Self-Doubt

I've been absolutely terrified every moment of my life...

— **Georgia O'Keeffe**

Befriending Fear

I owe you an apology. The quote above is a bit misleading. I quoted Ms. O'Keeffe accurately, but I left out the second half of the quote. I did this for effect. Without the second half, it's a wonderfully curious quote, given that it was spoken by an extraordinarily brave woman who was one of the greatest artists of the twentieth century. I've seen this quote appear this way in other texts, as well.

The vitally important second half of Ms. O'Keeffe's statement was this: "…and I've never let it keep me from doing a single thing I wanted to do." The second half completely alters the meaning and significance of the first half. I decided this would be a wonderful way to introduce a chapter that focuses on self-doubt.

Fear can be our friend. It's adaptive. It protects us from threats to our safety and happiness. Any medical procedure that intends to alter a patient's public presentation should arouse some concern in the patient. The questions, for our purposes, are these: how much concern is too much? And how do we manage our fears?

Befores and Afters

James was a funny guy. He used sarcasm a lot, and he found humor in some of the negative aspects of his life. During our initial session, he explained, "Some people believe if you don't have anything nice to say, you shouldn't say anything at all. I believe if you have only nice things to say, you're a liar—and you're boring. In other words, I'm the kind of guy who sees the bad in everything and everyone." He was joking—sort of.

James proudly labeled himself a cynic. A fifty-three-year-old model and actor, he had achieved a fair degree of success, typically playing handsome bad guys. He decided to undergo a cosmetic facial procedure. His goal was to preserve his vibrant appearance. It was very important to James that his face not look feminized or surgically altered.

He chose his surgeon carefully, and paid the full fee to reserve a date and secure his procedure. In the weeks after taking these decisive steps toward undergoing the procedure, he spent hours online, looking through dozens of before-and-after surgery photos on a daily basis. "It's become an obsession," he admitted in our first session. "That's really what led me to call you. My doctor suggested it. I don't know how to stop this. I'm freaking myself out."

"So, let me be sure I understand you, James. The surgeon you chose posted some photos of his work. You viewed them online, and the images concerned you?"

"Well, not exactly. My surgeon's photos looked good. The photos that concerned me are the ones from other doctors. I've seen some pretty gruesome stuff. Some people really get mangled."

It turned out James was looking at images of people whose procedures were not even performed by his doctor. He *was* looking up his chosen surgeon's before and after photos, but he was also searching for photos of any patients who had undergone the procedures he planned to undergo. "So," I asked, "can you put into words what you're looking for as you search through all of these photos?"

James eagerly replied, "Yes, as a matter of fact I can. I'm interested in learning and then memorizing the hundreds of ways idiots have ruined their faces with the very procedures I've selected. Smart, huh?"

This was one of the many moments when James used his sarcasm to let me know that he knew he was behaving in unkind ways toward himself.

"First, I want you to know I hear your sarcasm," I said. "And it's funny, but I think you and I also both know there's an aspect of it that isn't funny. I can help you with that. Let's examine what's happening. Essentially, you're concerned that your doctor will produce a result that looks like one of the ones you saw from other doctors?"

"Exactly. And I spoke with my doc about it," James said. "He said all the right things: different technique, different procedures, different recovery practices—I mean, all good answers. He told me all about his surgical technique. He explained that those surgeons were just not doing the procedure the way he does it, and he's way better."

"All of that sounds reassuring," I said, "but, from your tone, I gather you still don't feel reassured. Is that an accurate description?"

James leaned forward in his chair, as if to emphasize the following: "Exactly. I mean, accidents happen, right? And every body is unique, right? How can my doc really know my body will react the way it's supposed to? I mean, there could be an infection or an anesthetic error, or who knows what. I just feel like I'm not informed enough."

"You seem to focus a lot on complications and less likely outcomes."

James sat back on the couch and paused, looking confused and concerned. He sat quietly for a minute or so, slowly shaking his head as though he was silently repeating "no" to himself. He took a breath, looked up at me with a troubled expression, then said, in a tone entirely lacking humor or sarcasm, "The problem is, I can't pull the bad images out of my head. I just can't. I don't know what to do about it. I see them all the time, even in my sleep. It's freaking me out, and I'm afraid the damage is done. I can't forget them."

James's online research had sent him into a state of dread and self-doubt. He could only envision outcomes he wouldn't want. Once he chose his surgeon, his research should have been complete, but he couldn't allow himself to stop searching.

Anxiety, Self-Doubt, and the Desire for Control

James's excessive online research was a symptom of a larger issue. The psychotherapy with James needed to focus on his habitual tendency to freak himself out. This behavior didn't begin at age fifty-three. And it isn't something that was caused by some bad before-and-after images. James had been doing this, in different ways and to varying degrees, for much of his life.

"James, for us to move forward, it will help me to get to know how you handle certain situations," I said. "Can you tell me about your experience with auditions?"

"Well, the problem with auditions is you never know what they're looking for. You show up, you see a bunch of people there who look just like you, and you go in and you give them what you think they want, and then you leave. And you never really know what went wrong if you don't get the role."

"I understand. Can you tell me a little about how you prepare for auditions?"

James laughed. "Okay. Wait. This is funny. So, seriously, did my friend Susan call you and tell you to talk with me about this?"

"Nope. No contact with any Susan," I said.

James smiled, shook his head, quickly scratched behind his ear, and flicked his hair. These are the kinds of habitual actions therapists look for in initial sessions. Those kinds of simple movements often provide important unspoken information about a person's emotions. James then described his audition methods. "OK, well, I practice for hours. Days, when I have the time. Susan is an actress friend. We help each other with our auditions and audition tapes sometimes. The thing is, I've always been real detail-oriented. My procedure involves mapping out a bunch of different approaches to the scene—interpretations, I mean. And then I create a scheme for ranking them. That's how I choose the best interpretations."

"That's really elaborate," I said.

"Absolutely, but it's necessary. There are dozens of ways to play a scene. And you usually don't know exactly what they're looking for. You might make a single choice that they disagree with, and poof—you're gone. You just never know. It's a powerless feeling."

"Can you talk about the powerlessness?"

"It's crazymaking. Auditions are crazymaking. Sometimes I find myself pacing, playing out the possibilities in my mind, based on what I know about the casting director."

"Does online research sometimes give you some good information?"

"Who knows?" James replied. "I mean, maybe but maybe not. But I feel better if I know I gave it my all. In some ways, this is, like, the worst career a person like me could have chosen."

"Well, maybe. Maybe not," I said. "You know, it's interesting, in doing this work, I've realized it's actually pretty common for people to behave in similar ways in different parts of their lives. In your case, do you see a similarity between the really intense way you prepare for an audition and the way you approached researching 'before and after' images?"

"I didn't realize it, but yeah, in both situations I didn't want to feel out of control."

"Exactly. And I think we might get even more specific about it, James. In both situations, you seem to be striving for a degree of certainty that's unachievable."

"Well, I do see that," he replied. "I mean, I've always been someone who wanted predictability and security."

"And you chose a career that forces you to constantly confront the reality that you don't have complete control in life."

"Yeah, there's no doubt about that. I'm in a career that reminds me all the time that I don't have control. It's what I hate most about my career."

"And yet you chose it."

"What do you mean? I didn't choose *that* part?"

"This may sound strange, but I want to encourage you to be open to the idea that you did choose that."

"I chose to be miserable? What would I choose that?"

"Well," I said, "one way of looking at this is that our subconscious mind is always with us, influencing us. So, on a subconscious level, you may have chosen this career because, somewhere within you, you knew that you needed to find more tolerance with the uncertainties of life."

"Maybe." Then James added, "So, you think I busy myself beyond the point of it being helpful?"

"I do. It's really common in people who struggle with anxiety. We often feel anxious if we feel a lack of control in an important activity like an audition or a surgical procedure. Busying our mind distracts us from the reality of our lack of control. It's a way we sort of lie to ourselves. We make things seem more predictable and controllable."

"Okay. I get it, but I'm not sure what to do about that now, because I don't seem to be learning how to accept all of the powerlessness."

"I understand," I said. "There are methods for getting more comfortable with it. The fact that you recognize that this is a problem suggests you will likely be able to use the methods effectively."

When Low Self-Esteem Fuels Fear

James excelled at doubting himself. He practiced it often. To the outside world, he may have seemed self-assured and confident; a lot of habitually sarcastic people give this impression. But it's actually a self-protective posture. James tried to use the cynicism to manage his vulnerability. Unfortunately, cynicism is not a great choice as a coping strategy. It usually reinforces the vulnerability, and this is precisely the effect it had on James.

By compulsively checking online photos, James nurtured fears of surgical complications. The more he looked, the more he felt like maybe he had made a big mistake in choosing this procedure. His own research caused him to develop a lot of anxiety about it.

To understand why James would do this to himself, it's helpful to understand a little more about his personal history. James's childhood played a big role in his self-doubt. He was raised in rural Pennsylvania by his mother and stepfather after his father, Joe, died when James was five years old. Joe was an auto mechanic and, one day while Joe was lying under a car, the jack malfunctioned. The car fell on Joe, killing him instantly. James's mother remarried when James was seven. James acquired three half-siblings by the age of ten.

Most of the sarcasm went away when James described his childhood. He no longer seemed to be delivering one-liners. There was an authenticity in his presentation that he hadn't exhibited initially.

"My stepdad, Bill, was a property developer. He inherited money that he used to develop mobile home parks. He made a good living off of working-class people like my dad. That never sat well with me. He also took away my mom. And Bill never missed an opportunity to favor his kids over me. So, basically, Bill was a dick."

"It sounds like you didn't really feel like a part of the family once your mom married Bill."

"I always felt like a third wheel. Or a fifth wheel—an unnecessary wheel that got in the way."

"That's very sad, James. I'm sorry you went through that."

"It was tough," James said. "I was alone. Completely alone. I felt like my mom abandoned me. For years, I was mad at her too. But now I understand it better. I mean, from her perspective, she was lost when my dad died. It was the '60s, she was scraping by working at a diner. She didn't have any savings. She had nothing. And here comes this rich older guy who swept her away. Can't blame her, really."

"And she started a family with him, and you felt like an intruder?"

"Right away. That's how it was. That's why I left at seventeen." James shook his head. "I couldn't wait to get away. I washed dishes at that same diner my mom had worked at, and I saved enough money to buy a bus ticket to LA. I packed an old suitcase my mom had, got a seat against the window in the last row of the bus, and turned on my cassette of 'Jet Airliner' by the Steve Miller Band." James scratched behind his ear, flicked his hair, and laughed out loud at this memory. "I think I listened to that song a thousand times between Pennsylvania and California. Right out of a Hollywood screenplay."

"That's such a vivid description. Right down to the music. You were really courageous," I said.

"Yeah, the courage of a seventeen-year-old, right?" James smiled. I could see the wheels in his head turning. I knew he had more to say. And as the wheels turned, I could see his smile fading. When he continued, he was speaking not as a fifty-three-year-old admiring his seventeen-year-old self, but as a fifty-three-year-old who has learned things from life that the seventeen-year-old hadn't yet been taught. "I feel like courage grows until about nineteen," he said, "That's when life starts chipping away at it. That's what it feels like to me, anyway. The older you get, the more opportunities you have to see the consequences of screwing up."

When James spoke more about his childhood, his self-doubt made complete sense. First, he had always felt like he was on his own in the world. He also described feeling like he could never do anything right in his stepdad's eyes. Though he hated to admit it, Bill's dismissive behavior deeply damaged James.

Unfortunately, when James left Pennsylvania with only a single suitcase, he brought his self-esteem issue with him. That issue led James to continually test himself. Whenever he performed well, he would feel relieved. When he committed an error of some kind, it would reactivate that inner belief that he was the boy Bill had rejected. That he was just not good enough. This is why he became so fearful of failing. To James, failure meant confirmation of his inadequacy. This is why powerlessness felt much more threatening to James than it would to most people. His self-esteem rested on every risk he ever took.

This dynamic is especially dangerous for a patient preparing for cosmetic surgery. As I had previously mentioned to him, those procedures never come with a guarantee. To cope well before and after them, the patient has to tolerate a lot of uncertainty. One way to do this is to trust the surgeon. For someone like James, who tends to distrust most people, trusting his surgeon was not going to be easy.

At my urging, James agreed to use his psychotherapy to explore his trust issues. He started by carefully examining the accuracy of any bits and pieces of distrust he held toward his surgeon. This is a type of work psychologists call "cognitive restructuring." I also encouraged James to discuss examples of distrust he felt toward other people. We used these examples to practice testing the accuracy of the thoughts he relied on to preserve his cynicism and distrust.

James and I also needed to work on raising his self-esteem. He needed to honor his decisions so he would not be as inclined to abuse himself if the outcome was less than he'd hoped for. Improved self-esteem would likely help him learn to trust himself enough to cope with whatever outcomes he encountered in life.

Perfectionism and Low Self-Esteem

To improve his self-confidence, James had to see the ways he contributed to his own sense of inadequacy. I administered a brief psychological test to him. The test is well-validated and brief. It is not available to the general public. It assesses a person's comfort level with uncertainty, and I sometimes use this test with cosmetic surgery patients. Not surprisingly, James's responses indicated he was very uncomfortable with uncertainty.

James engaged in a lot of perfectionistic behaviors that were aimed at eliminating all uncertainty. Most perfectionists don't realize how demoralizing perfectionism is. Perfectionism is the opposite of a strategy for feeling confident. In our unpredictable world populated by inherently imperfect humans, perfectionism is destined to fail. So, on a personal level, perfectionism engenders feelings of inadequacy in the person exhibiting it.

Habits are always hard to change. With someone like James, helping him to change his habitual perfectionism was going to be particularly difficult. First, he felt more comfortable being that way. He'd been doing it for years. But there was a deeper psychological issue that added to the difficulty. The underlying issue tying James to his perfectionism was that, ironically, this way of being maintained his sense of inadequacy.

I'm not suggesting James consciously sought to feel inadequate, or that he enjoyed it. Like most perfectionistic thinkers, James's perfectionism was an unconscious method of self-sabotage. And he was committed to preserving the self-image of someone who was lacking. His therapy needed to address this sense of personal inadequacy. Perfectionism fuels and perpetuates self-doubt. These qualities had become fundamental aspects of his identity.

Managing Self-Doubt to Maximize Your Cosmetic Success

James was addicted to continually mulling over past mistakes and worry-ing about future ones. Psychologists who study the tendency to rumi-nate in these ways have found that rumination is often a precursor to depression. Rumination can fuel depression and depression, in turn, can strengthen the tendency to ruminate. The classic rabbit hole.

Rumination is particularly destructive because it tends to be self-per-petuating. It's often all-consuming. For James, rumination blocked him from engaging in healthy problem-solving behaviors, keeping him stuck, forever spinning his wheels. This activated his anxiety and made him more vulnerable to developing depression.

Cosmetic surgery patients often engage in this kind of behavior. There is so much uncertainty when a patient is preparing for or healing from these procedures. Old habits like the tendency to ruminate often emerge, particularly during stressful periods. The consequence is unnecessary and counterproductive stress.

The alternative to rumination is a more self-compassionate way of treating oneself. Rumination is a form of self-punishment. This is true whether our thoughts are directed at ourselves or at those who have wronged us. Rumination is a rejection of what is. In this sense, it is self-defeating. We need to find ways to accept the things that exist, even if we don't like some of them.

James' rumination revealed his intolerance for dissatisfaction. Life sends undesirable things to us sometimes. It's inevitable. People who ruminate tend to focus too much on the things they got but hadn't wanted. Instead of practicing acceptance of what is, they engage in a perpetual and desperate effort to eliminate all of the unpleasant experiences. Of course, it's an impossible task—but it's addictive. It's very difficult for them to resist engaging in the effort.

Habitual Dissatisfaction, Fear, and Your Cosmetic Procedure

James's decision to direct sarcasm toward the world revealed his habitual struggle with dissatisfaction. His sarcasm communicated that nothing is worth respecting. The disrespect was his way of detaching from other people and systems while communicating his expectation that they would fail him. Predictably, his attitude played a role in the way the world reacted to him. People are less likely to engage closely with someone who communicates disrespect and disinterest in them. So, James unwittingly played a role in causing his world to seem less friendly and helpful than it otherwise might have.

His cynicism was a defense, an effort to protect himself from feeling like a failure, if he ever were to fail. It was the old "I wasn't really trying" defense. We all have used it, sometimes intentionally, sometimes not. But deep down, James didn't attribute failures to not trying. Like a lot of people who habitually rely on sarcasm, deep down, James normally attributed failures to his own inadequacy.

Behind the humor, James was reacting to the world in much the same way he learned to react in his childhood. He felt alone and vulnerable. He felt as though he didn't have anyone to rely on other than himself. This made decisions terrifying. If decisions were to lead to unpleasant consequences, he had no one to help him clean up the messes.

In this way, James never fully recovered from the emotional injuries he suffered as a child. This is what I meant when I said he would say things in a joking way, sort of. Underneath his sarcasm was a mix of fear and disappointment that was not funny at all to James.

James's cynical tendency to feel dissatisfied was especially important to address within the context of his upcoming surgery. We all know people who live by the adage "expect the worst and hope for the best." James was one of those people. People like James fear dissatisfaction so much that they choose to expect it in the hope that they will feel better prepared for it. Their hope is to lessen their disappointment in the face of dissatisfaction.

For a cosmetic patient, there are at least two problems with this way of thinking. First, fearing dissatisfaction so intensely can cause a patient to avoid engaging fully in the healing process. Particularly in the initial phase of recovery, cosmetic patients need to vigilantly follow their doctor's guidelines, actively monitoring and treating their wounds to promote proper healing.

The problem is, the patient is not at their best immediately after a surgical procedure. The initial phases of recovery can be very difficult. There can be a lot of swelling, pain, and other unpleasant bodily reactions such as bleeding. If a patient finds the prospect of an undesirable outcome completely intolerable, the patient may withdraw, fearing the worst. This diminished motivation and ostrich-head-buried-in-the-sand approach can lead to poor management of wounds. This is a common way the patient's negligence can end up diminishing the success of a cosmetic outcome.

The second problem a cosmetic procedure patient confronts, if they have an excessive fear of dissatisfaction, was actually articulated by James once, when he said, "I got to a point, looking at before and after photos, where I could not tell the difference. And you know what? They all looked terrible! I could find flaws in all of them. I found myself questioning what the hell I was doing by having this procedure!" In other words, his fear of disappointment could cause him to demand a very narrow, perfectionistic outcome, thereby ensuring his disappointment.

When James would view before and after photos, he was engaging in an unhealthy form of rehearsal. He was gaining experience applying his perfectionistic views onto surgical outcomes. In other words, without realizing it, he was practicing feeling disappointed. Not a great way to prepare for a cosmetic surgical procedure.

The kind of black-and-white thinking James often relied on is common among overly picky people. Black-and-white thinking refers to seeing things with less complexity than they deserve, as either entirely good or entirely bad, for instance. In reality, most things in life fall within the gray zone.

The tendency to fear dissatisfaction can be diminished if black-and-white thinking is reduced. This is a vitally important issue for any cosmetic surgery patient to address, and they can do it with the help of effective psychotherapy. The good news is that this does not require the patient to dramatically alter their perceptions. On the contrary, the objective is simply to embrace a broader definition of surgical success.

Cosmetic outcomes are always uncertain. Patients need to be prepared to accept a less-than-perfect outcome. If they can, they are more capable of embracing the reality that risk is unavoidable in any surgical intervention, and particularly in a cosmetic one.

Developing Internal Acceptance to Cope with Uncertainty

Mindfulness meditation is sometimes thought of as a way a person becomes friendlier with themself. There is a close compatibility between Western psychotherapy and mindfulness. Both traditions place great value on treating a person with unconditional compassion, respect, and friendliness. Both mindfulness and Western psychotherapy encourage people to treat themselves as they would treat a close friend. Another way of saying this is that in both traditions, we imagine there is a supportive friend with us—inside us—every moment of our lives.

Like a lot of people, James behaved in ways that added to the struggles that life sent him. This is one of the ways a person can be "their own worst enemy." For people who treat themselves this way, I suggest an exercise called the Wise and Supportive Inner Friend Exercise. Two core ideas underlie this exercise. First, people often use their mind to evaluate themselves in ways that are unkind, even abusive. Sometimes this is referred to as the "critical voice" inside us. Second, we tend to be nicer to ourselves when we are with a supportive friend.

This exercise involves practicing seeing yourself as never alone. You are always with a friend who supports you unconditionally. The point of the exercise is to practice hearing the difference between the way you tend to treat yourself and the way a person who unconditionally accepts you would treat you. This exercise had a noticeable impact on James.

Exercise: The Wise and Supportive Inner Friend Voice

In your journal, create a table with three columns. Label the left column "Description of an unpleasant situation." Label the second column "My reaction to that situation." Label the third column "My close friend's supportive reaction." This is a thought exercise so the content of any of the columns can be real or imagined. The objective is to explore the ways you tend to treat yourself and the degree to which your treatment of yourself resembles the way you would expect a supportive friend to treat you.

Description of a real or imagined unpleasant situation.	My reaction to that situation.	My close friend's supportive reaction.

This exercise can be repeated for multiple experiences. It's best to try to be completely honest when constructing the message of the critical inner voice. It's helpful to look over your work after completing it. Sit with the results. Try to notice themes in the ways you treat yourself, such as the things you tend to focus on. Try to be curious about the differences between your words and the friend's words. Consider practicing this exercise several times each week.

**Exercise: The Wise and Supportive Inner Friend Voice,
Cosmetic Surgery Version**

A separate version of this exercise focuses, in particular, on the experience of undergoing a cosmetic procedure. In this version, the left column is labeled "Description of feared surgical outcome." The second column is labeled "My reaction if I were to have that outcome." The third column is labeled "My friend's supportive and encouraging reaction to the outcome."

More Exercises!

The following several exercises were helpful to James. I include them because, if you struggle in ways that resemble how James struggled, they may benefit you, too. These three wise inner friend exercises are all particularly helpful for people who tend to doubt their own perceptions and conclusions.

 **Exercise: Manage the Dosage:
Fearful Thoughts Medicine**

This is a simple behavioral practice with one basic objective: to limit how much you think about fears. The idea is, thinking about something we fear is like medicine. It's good to take that medicine, sometimes. It helps us feel safe. But even good medicine is bad for us if we overdose on it. So this exercise helps us "dose" ourselves on the medicine of fearful thoughts.

1. First, schedule a time each day when you will permit
    yourself to think about your fears. Maybe you will want
    to journal about them at the scheduled time. You may
    need more time in the first week, so schedule about an
    hour for you to think and write about your fears. Be
    specific; say, from 5:00 p.m. to 6:00 p.m. In the second
    week, decrease the time by fifteen minutes.

2. During the day, walk around with a small notepad, or
    your phone. When you think of a worry you have, write
    it down or create a note in your phone. Be as brief as
    possible. Then go back to your day.

3. At the scheduled time, honor your agreement with
    yourself. Go to a quiet place, pull out your notes,
    and write and/or think about them. The objective in
    thinking about them is to identify them very clearly. In
    other parts of this book, you will learn techniques for
    assessing the accuracy of the fearful thoughts. You may
    want to use those exercises here as well.

4. Integrate the "Stop It" technique. During the day, if
    your mind focuses on a fear you already had written
    down, literally say to yourself "stop it" as a way of
    telling yourself to stop thinking about it. You might
    also do a brief meditation for a minute or so to help you
    refocus on your breaths and then on whatever you were
    doing. This can help you let go of the thoughts and
    return to your daily activity.

By helping you to manage what your brain focuses on throughout the day, this exercise is all about helping you to assert your authority over your brain. Your brain is a tool. You own that tool and you get to decide when and how you choose to use it.

One thing I've already told you bears repeating: managing your thoughts isn't easy. Try to be patient with yourself. All people need to practice this to become proficient. Hopefully, you can see how well this fits with the mindfulness meditation practice. Both practices are aimed at being more mindful. In this way, they both help us learn to better manage our thoughts, feelings, and behaviors.

Fear Paralysis

The next exercise focuses on managing fear. One way psychologists help people manage their fears is by helping them practice not giving fear the power to alter behavior. There is a good reason for doing this. Research suggests most of the things we fear either never happen or happen in a form that is not nearly as bad as we feared. One reason overly anxious people experience functional problems is that they tend to overestimate the likelihood of bad things happening. A related second reason is that they too often allow their actions to be altered by their fears. This is why there is a simple practice that people with anxiety are often encouraged to adopt: *feel the fear and do it anyway.*

Note that this is not a practice to be used when we see clear evidence of danger. For instance, this practice is inappropriate when considering crossing a busy street with a blindfold on. This practice is for the times when we feel anxious that an undesirable thing that we can cope with might occur despite there being no convincing evidence that it likely will occur.

You can probably see the relevance of this to surgical procedures. Sometimes we benefit in life by taking risks. A patient preparing for a cosmetic procedure might fear there will be a complication despite the reality that a complication is highly unlikely. Or, a patient may fear a bad outcome even though it's not at all likely that any outcome would be so bad that it could not be addressed later in a corrective procedure. This is not to say any risk is worth taking, but rather that a patient who is unwilling to take a risk is likely to act against their best interests. The point is we benefit if we overcome a knee-jerk tendency to always alter our behavior in the face of fear.

The reason this exercise is helpful is simple: we rarely do something well without practice. This exercise gives us practice acting in the face of fear. Doing the following exercise regularly will improve your ability to tolerate the unpleasantness of risk-taking. In so doing, you will reduce your discomfort with uncertainty and will undergo any cosmetic service with more confidence in your strength and resilience.

 Exercise: Feel the Fear and Proceed Anyway

In your journal, copy the table reproduced below. You will create a table with seven columns. Label the left (first) column "Action I Fear Taking." Label the second column "Feared Consequence." Label the third column "Likelihood Rating (0–100)." In this column, give your best estimate of the likelihood the feared consequence will occur (0 = impossible, 100 = certain). Label the fourth column "Possible Desired Consequences." List as many possible desired consequences as you can think of. Label the fifth column "Likelihood Rating (0–100)." In this column, rate the likelihood each desired consequence will occur. If you have more than one desired consequence, write down a rating for each. Label the sixth column "Reward." In this column, describe what you will give yourself as a reward for taking the risk and doing what you identified in the first column. Label the seventh column "Actual Consequence." In this column briefly describe the true consequence that happened if you did the thing identified in the first column. If you did not do the thing identified in column one, leave the seventh column blank.

You can see an example on the next page:

Action I Fear Taking	Feared Consequence	Likelihood Rating (0–100)	Possible Desired Consequences	Likelihood Rating (0–100)	Reward	Actual Consequence
Dancing at friend's wedding.	I will be look foolish and be mocked.	50	I will feel like part of the party rather than a wallflower.	90	I will allow myself a piece of cake.	I did not notice any mockery and I had fun.
Going out in public when I look bad.	People will stare. I will feel humiliated.	70	I will feel less dependent on others' approval.	80	I will buy myself a foot massage.	Some looked, I think. But doing this makes me stronger.

The value of this exercise is it gives you the opportunity to remind yourself that life is unpredictable. When we allow our fears to dictate our behaviors, we are assuming that we can predict the consequences of actions more accurately than we actually can. This is a cognitive exercise because it focuses on improving your thinking. The goal is not so much to tell you what you should do, but rather to remind you that any decision involves risk, to help you begin to embrace that reality, and to factor the awareness of it into your behavior choices.

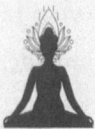

Exercise: Mindfulness Meditation for Befriending Your Emotions

Reminder: a guided version of this meditation is located at DrAlanGoodwin.com

This is a mindfulness meditation that provides practice coexisting with all of your emotions.

1. Find a quiet, private place where you can practice staying present.

2. Assume a comfortable, relaxed position. You can sit or lie down, but it's best to remain awake. Choose a position that will enable you to remain alert, but not stiff or tense.

3. Breathe. Stop. Be. Just take slow, deep breaths in and out.

4. Notice whatever your five senses reveal to you. Take your time. As you breathe, identify any smells, sights, sounds, tastes, or things you are touching.

5. Continue to breathe slowly and deeply. If you can, exhale a bit longer than you inhale. Focus on your breathing. Try to maintain this focus. If you notice your mind wandering, gently remind yourself to return your focus to your breaths. Remember: this is difficult. Try to allow that.

6. As you breathe, notice any emotions within yourself. Whatever the emotion, focus on it. Try to be curious

about it. Imagine you are a research scientist studying emotion in a laboratory and your own body is your specimen. Observe and note any emotion that occurs to you as you continue to focus on your breath. Slow, comfortable breaths, in and out. Also notice any physical feelings that accompany the emotion. Consciously remain present with these sensations. If you notice yourself trying to push a sensation away, gently refocus on your breathing and allow the sensation to coexist with you. View the sensations with interest and curiosity.

7. Notice how your emotions evolve as you observe them. Try not to censor yourself. Treat every emotion as important. Try not to judge any of them.

8. Return your focus to your breath. Continue to breathe slowly and deeply. If you can, exhale a bit longer than you inhale.

9. Now use your breath to help you bring to yourself the feeling of self-compassion. Notice that this work is difficult. Acknowledge that you are persevering in spite of the difficulty.

10. Finally, use your breath to help you bring yourself in contact with the feeling of gratitude. As you breathe, quietly say to yourself, "I am grateful to be sitting with my emotions." Repeat that sentence. Notice that you are able to do this meditation. Try to feel thankful for that. Sit in gratitude while focusing on your breath. Repeat the sentence as many times as you'd like.

11. As you continue to focus on your breathing, you may notice other emotions within you. Try to remain present with any emotion you perceive. Remember: you can feel negative emotions and still welcome gratitude. If you notice yourself pushing negative emotions away, accept that, then try to return your focus to your breath.

12. Take a few moments to empower yourself as you breathe. Use mantras to remind yourself that you are coping. Choose a mantra that is brief, positive, accurate, and empowering. A few examples: "I am coping." "I am strong." "I am blessed." "I am healing." "I am improving." "I am committed." "Struggles are opportunities."

There is no minimum time for this exercise. Your practice session can be as brief as one minute, or as long as thirty minutes to an hour. Whatever the length, put forth a sincere effort. Above all, have patience with the process. This is a skill. Skills develop over time. It's best to begin to practice this exercise long before your planned procedure. In this way, you will begin your practice of focusing on body sensations when the context is an absence of pain. Remember that the key to this exercise is staying present. Practice remaining present with your body.

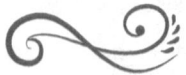

CHAPTER 7

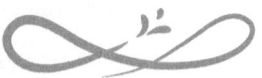

Hidden In Plain Sight: Ubiquitous, Intrusive Anxiety

What one dreads, one must see.

—Japanese Proverb

Ubiquitous Anxiety

We have discussed the simple definition of anxiety as a fear that something may happen that will cause sadness. We feel many kinds of anxiety—social anxiety, evaluation anxiety, and test anxiety, to name only a few. In this chapter, we will explore some of the ways cosmetic patients struggle with anxiety, both before and after the procedure. And we will explore the ways patients can confront and overcome those struggles.

Julie's Intimidation

Julie struck terror into other people. Not because she was fighting a potentially disfiguring form of cancer. The cancer had not yet disfigured her, so that wasn't what made Julie such a scary person. She was just scary. That's the way she explained it, anyway. But I'm getting ahead of myself.

Julie first learned of the cancer when she was thirty-six years old. She was a bright, active, and attractive marketing executive. She sought psychotherapy to cope with anxiety while preparing for a second surgical procedure. The first surgery had been unsuccessful. She was confronting the possibility that, in the second surgery, parts of her face might need to be removed to save her life.

Julie was a lifelong social activist. She began assuming leadership roles in high school. When we met, Julie was advancing in her marketing career while, in her spare time, playing an active role in her community, organizing protests, environmental cleanups, and fundraisers serving various causes.

In our first session, Julie described her difficulty in this way:

"I know I've been very lucky. I've never confronted the issues so many people struggle with. I've been healthy psychologically, I never had weight issues, I never had any serious medical issues, and I met a man who loves me very much. And now he reassures me on a daily basis that he'll stand by me no matter what happens to my appearance."

She explained she underwent an initial surgical procedure to eliminate the condition. The procedure failed. This meant that both her health and her appearance remained under threat by the cancer. She needed another procedure.

Her medical condition was frightening. Anyone in Julie's condition would benefit from strengthened coping skills to persevere through her difficult journey. But that wasn't exactly why she sought my help. The unusual thing about Julie was the psychological issue she wanted to address. "I believe the first surgical procedure failed because of me," she said. "That may sound crazy, but I'm convinced it's true. As you'll see, I'm a very assertive person. I intimidate people."

I replied, "First, Julie, I want you to know I'm glad to hear that you assert yourself to get your needs met. That will be a great resource in our work together. And, although this may sound strange, I'm actually glad to know that you feel like you need to protect people from that quality in you. That's a valuable insight into how you see yourself. But I do want to request something. I want to ask you to please let me know if you're ever feeling the need to protect me from you. Will you commit to doing that?"

"Yes, I can do that," she replied.

"And I mean from any part of you," I continued. "Your assertiveness, your feelings, the things you say, your facial expressions—anything. Do you know why I'm asking this of you?"

"I think so," Julie said. "I guess you want to know when I'm judging myself."

"That's not what I meant, but that's really insightful. I agree that when you're protecting me from you, you're judging yourself, and we should examine it when that happens. What I had in mind was that your protection of me is a gift to me. I want to encourage you not to give me that gift or any gift, for that matter. You and I are embarking on a relationship. But, unlike any other relationship you have in your life, in this one you don't give. You only receive. It's a strange thing, but it's the foundation of psychotherapy. So I want you to know that my goal will be to help you to stop giving me the gift of protecting me from you."

Sometimes people listen, but they don't seem to be hearing the message well. Julie listened and heard. After I finished, she replied, "Thank you. I had never thought of psychotherapy in that way. I understand, and I appreciate your saying what you said."

"You're welcome. So, now that we're past that, I want to pick up on something you said earlier. You said you feel responsible for the first surgical procedure's outcome. Can you say more about that?"

Julie responded in a casual way that seemed to communicate there was no question that her perception was accurate. "Sure. When I met with my surgeon, I told her it was very important that she not do anything that would cause people to detect that I had surgery." Julie finished that sentence and then stopped. I was waiting for her to continue, but she said nothing more.

"Did you feel like it was unreasonable for you to have said that to the surgeon?"

Again, her response was prompt and confident. "Unreasonable? No. Dumb? Without question. When I say things, people feel boxed in. I've been told that a thousand times. I am absolutely sure my intensity led her and the surgical oncologist to operate in overly conservative ways. And now my condition is worse."

I continued to seek clarification from Julie. I knew I needed to remain mindful of how steadfast she was. I knew she wasn't going to change her mind right away. But I wanted to gather information about what led her to believe she was responsible. "That last detail was helpful, Julie. I want to be sure I'm understanding it, though. You're saying you had two surgeons for your procedure, right?"

"Yes."

"Okay, so my understanding is that, in situations like yours, there is a surgical oncologist and a separate cosmetic surgeon. Is that right?"

"Yes, that's right," Julie replied.

"Did either of those specialist surgeons tell you they altered their surgical practices because of your cosmetic concerns?"

"No, they didn't."

"We're talking about a very serious pair of procedures, performed by two surgeons who each had extensive specialized training and experience. And you're concerned that they both were intimidated from doing their best work?" I asked.

"My husband, Ken, says he's at his wits' end with me. He says I'm crazy to be worried about this. He actually thinks it's sexist of me because both surgeons are women. I think that's ridiculous. But anyway, I'm convinced I altered their work."

At this point, I felt the need to back off. I didn't want my protectiveness of Julie to turn into something that might have felt to her like an attack. "I understand. And, Julie, this isn't an inquisition. Our goal isn't to find answers to every question. Our job together is to explore who you are and how that might impact the patterned ways you think, feel, and behave. It's vitally important to me that you feel safe talking about whatever perceptions or fears or other thoughts or feelings you have."

I stopped, giving Julie time to sit with those words. After sitting a moment, she leaned forward and took a Kleenex. She neatly folded it three times and then gently but firmly pressed it against the inside corner of each of her eyes. She sniffled softly and then continued in a tone that reflected more vulnerability. "I feel very responsible. I wasn't trusting them. I should have trusted my surgeons. I shouldn't have been my normal over-controlling self. It's just that, the truth is, deep down, these operations terrify me."

"You say that as though you shouldn't have felt fearful. Do you feel that way?"

"I'm not sure how I feel about my fear. But I know I need to stop dealing with it by turning everyone around me into a marionette."

"I see your strength, Julie. You're a smart, assertive woman. That's clear the minute you speak. But I'm interested in how much power you believe you have over other people. I'm eager to learn more about that, and also more about how hard you are on yourself."

"I believe in accountability," Julie replied. "I have more surgeries ahead. I need help letting go of control so I don't screw up another procedure."

"I understand. I think I can help you reduce the controlling behaviors. The first step toward achieving that is going to involve giving voice to your anxiety. Can we do that now? Can you tell me about the visions and thoughts a second procedure conjure up in you?"

"Well, without going into the details, I fear if it fails, I will be disfigured. I'll be someone people gawk at. That would certainly alter my consulting work. It's possible more surgeries could correct the issues, but there are no guarantees. I also envision people pitying me. I'm not sure that's better than being stared at in horror. I just feel like I'll never be able to ignore it and live a normal life."

Blaming and Shaming and Why Bad Things Really Happen

Julie and I set specific goals for her psychotherapy. Some of the work, of course, involved exploring her fears and creating a safe space where she could talk about and feel her sadness about her serious medical condition. We devoted time to grieving the loss of her health and to exploring the newfound distrust of her body. She embraced health behaviors over which she had control, and acceptance of the things over which she had less or no control.

She also struggled with the fear that she might regain her health but lose her attractiveness. She had never been a person who derived self-respect based solely on her beauty. Still, the thought of losing it was causing unfamiliar feelings of self-doubt. As she described it, "I find myself fearing that, without my looks, I won't know how to function in the world. It feels overwhelming."

For our purposes, I want to focus this discussion on the work Julie and I did together related to her sense of responsibility for the failed first procedure. We agreed there would be two aspects of this work. First, we would discuss the procedure together in more detail. Second, I asked Julie to speak with both surgeons separately, and to ask each one whether her concerns altered the surgical decisions. She agreed to do this.

Not surprisingly, Julie's surgeons each denied that her concerns altered their work in any way. They explained the medical reasons why the first surgical procedure did not eliminate the condition. Julie felt convinced by the surgeons' explanations and their insistence that none of the three of them were to blame. The surgeons both explained to Julie that there were reasons why the procedures were simply not effective at that time.

When I asked Julie whether she felt relieved, she said, "Actually, strangely enough, I don't feel relieved. Not at all, really. I can't tell you why. In a sense I'm baffled by how I feel. But it just feels unsatisfying."

I wasn't surprised to hear this. Julie was struggling with something that's actually very common but not well-understood by most people. Even plenty of mental health professionals don't really address the issue at the core of Julie's fear and sense of responsibility. "This may sound convoluted," I said, "but bear with me. There's a well-known psychological preference for explanations that all humans have. In fact, we prefer an explanation for why an unhappy event occurs even if the explanation is divorced from reality. So, for instance, psychological studies have confirmed that people feel relief if they attribute a sad event like a car crash to something like a curse, or astrology, or karma. Do you have any idea why this would be so?"

"No," Julie said. "I mean, I think curses are silly. I would never think a curse caused something."

"Okay, but thinking more broadly about what any explanation provides, the idea is, life is unpredictable, and that scares us. The fears we feel are expressed in our anxiety. Anxiety indicates that we perceive a danger. At one time, the dangers were threats from animals or rival tribes. Today, the threats that fuel our anxiety are things like car crashes and robberies. The point is, we use our anxiety to try to see those things coming before they kill us. So, our anxiety helps us to feel safer. If I know to look out for lions, I feel a bit safer from the lions. Does that make sense?"

"It does. But I don't know what this has to do with me. I don't feel particularly safe these days."

"Well, from the anxious person's perspective, anxiety seems to enhance predictability. Predictability gives us a sense of control, which helps us feel safer. So, if a bad thing happens and we can blame someone for it—let's say, you—for the failed first procedure, you will feel some comfort because it enables you to believe 'Okay, so as long as I don't screw up again by pressuring the doctors, this thing won't happen again.' Blaming yourself enables you to indulge the fiction that you have control over the outcome. And that feels reassuring. I think this is why you blamed yourself, Julie. It gave you the impression that you can make things go better next time. People do this to themselves all the time—because we want to believe we can prevent bad things from happening."

"But I don't feel reassured," Julie replied. "If that's why I did it, why would I still feel unsatisfied?"

"You feel unsatisfied because, on some level, you know you're not to blame."

Julie sat with this thought for a moment. Then she said, "That provides some comfort, but I'm feeling kind of empty. I don't know what to do. Am I supposed to just float through life until the operation?"

"There's plenty you can do to cope. Now that we can let go of the need to blame you for the first procedure's outcome, we can focus our work on helping you enter the next procedure with a healthy mindset. You and I will work on helping you accept the limited control you have over the outcome. You do have some control, just not as much as you thought, and not in the way you thought. That's where our focus should be."

"Well, if you want a good laugh, call Ken and tell him you're planning to get me to stop pretending to be in control of the world. It'll be the best laugh he's had in weeks."

Julie laughed, but then stopped suddenly and began to cry. Through her tears, she said, "This last six months has been so hard on Ken. I've been all over the place. Angry one minute, bawling my eyes out the next minute. I chew him out when he makes the slightest mistake. And he's been an angel. He never attacks back. He is so strong. He's always there. People think I'm always in charge. For the past six months, I've felt out of my mind. Everyone sees him as this nice guy who follows a few steps behind me and does what I say. The truth is, I've been relying on him since the beginning. And in the last six months, I've just felt so scared and lost."

"I'm so glad you have each other. It sounds like a beautiful partnership."

"I'm very lucky," Julie said.

"And I'm really glad you allowed yourself to say and feel those things here, Julie. I think one of the things we can work on is helping you to be gentle with yourself. I hope you'll be able to use this space however you think will be most helpful on a given day. I want you to know that I'll be trying to help create that kind of a space for you."

Meditation and Gratitude

In our initial sessions, Julie repeatedly noted she had always felt too independent to benefit from psychotherapy. Contrary to her expectations, her independence was a great asset in her therapy. The same courage and non-defensiveness that enabled her to speak to me so frankly also helped her look carefully at herself. When she did that, she saw how often she felt the need to feel in control in her life. And she was willing to examine that.

One of the main objectives in our work was to help Julie utilize mindfulness and meditation to acquire a different relationship with the outer world. There was a very real possibility that, after the surgical procedure, Julie would encounter a world that would see her completely differently than before. Julie had always been a dynamo and a social magnet. How would she engage in a world that, upon first seeing her, might not feel drawn to her? For instance, she wondered whether her wit and playfulness would be dimmed if she were viewed differently. We explored issues like these, and she also used a daily meditation practice to sit with these and other thoughts and concerns.

Julie worked hard, both within the psychotherapy and during the time between our sessions. She also increased the frequency of her yoga practice. She was so open to the work. She told me she had never meditated prior to our discussions, yet she was willing to implement two different meditations. She did a daily mindfulness meditation, as well as a Tonglen meditation three to four times each week (reproduced at the end of Chapter 4).

Between the meditation work and her work in therapy, Julie quieted her need for control. Coincidentally, she also became active in Al-Anon, for reasons unrelated to her medical situation. During her therapy, she often discussed the intersection between the psychotherapy and the Al-Anon work, such as the serenity prayer. That prayer reminds us to see and accept the things over which we have limited or no control, such as how other people react to us.

Julie's Outcome

In the end, Julie's story had the happiest of endings—or new beginnings. Julie's second surgical procedure was successful. The concerns she felt about becoming disfigured resolved over time, after a series of cosmetic interventions. Her worst cosmetic fears were not realized because the procedures resurrected her appearance to an astounding degree. Still, she needed to persevere through that process, and she did it beautifully.

Julie's strength, humor, and insight were all put to good use. She needed to cope with a scary series of surgical procedures. Although Julie didn't end up needing to establish a new relationship between herself and the outer world, she did it anyway. She reported feeling more in touch with her sense of gratitude and less fearful of the things over which she had limited control.

Julie also found herself more connected to other people. She said her awareness of her own struggle caused her to feel much more compassion in her daily life. Julie's transformation was beautiful to witness. I saw the changes in our sessions. Julie was always a lovely person, but she acquired a warm and inviting quality that she didn't have when she was so focused on maintaining control over everything in her life.

Julie's cosmetic issues had threatened her career. She needed to confront those fears and cope with the risk that her professional and personal lives might have changed dramatically, after the procedure. Cosmetic patients often confront these kinds of fears, but sometimes the fears differ from what they first seem to be. Sometimes other issues hide behind the cosmetic concerns. This will be the subject of the next section.

Cosmetic Surgery and Career Preservation

Perhaps the most descriptive way to refer to Glen is that he reminded me of an older version of Ryan Seacrest. He presented impressively. He was a handsome, energetic fifty-eight-year-old advertising executive. He had an athletic though not overly muscular physique. It was easy to see why Glen was successful in advertising. He exuded enthusiasm that was infectious and reflected a kind of natural youthfulness.

When I discussed aging with Glen, he was direct and non-defensive. "I do feel younger than what society seems to think a fifty-eight-year-old should be. And yet I still feel the pressure to remain youthful. Living in Los Angeles, near the beach, and working in a youth-dominated field, it's hard to ignore that pressure. This is especially true in my field." Glen explained that people in advertising need to feel "connected." "We need to know current trends and be able to predict future ones. Sometimes we need to create future trends. And young people lead the way. So, you need to be connected to them. In advertising, youth represents relevancy. Advertising executives who lose their relevancy get cut by the firm."

Glen was an engaging and interesting guy. Raised in a middle-class home in New Jersey, he graduated from New York University and took a job with a Manhattan-based advertising firm. He quickly distinguished himself in that office, assuming a leadership position. Eventually he was recruited by a Los Angeles firm, where he continued to thrive. He served on various boards and was an active supporter of the arts and of organizations that addressed animal and environmental welfare.

"Service seems to be very important to you," I said to him once.

He replied without hesitation, "Absolutely. I was raised in the Catholic church and I attended Catholic schools. The nuns taught me the value of service."

Sometimes, when a prospective cosmetic patient comes to see me, the client's needs are clear from the initial session. On many occasions, the focus of our work emerges after some period of time. Glen was an example of the latter kind of client. We really only defined our work after we began exploring his family history. It was during this exploration process that I asked, "Can you say more about the role service has played in your personal growth and development?"

This seemed to energize him. He sat up, leaned forward in the armchair, and said, as if there could only be this answer, "Oh, I'm a completely different person because of service. Completely. Helping people in rural locations who have so little, or animals that are struggling just to survive, you can't return from that being the same person you were."

"Can you say more about how that service work changed you?" I asked.

"In so many ways. I don't think we can be truly healthy unless we serve others. I think this is true for everyone. I have been so insanely lucky in my life. Loving parents, a secure home, a safe community—each of those is a tremendous blessing. Service helps me to remember my gratitude every day. Every day I remind myself of that."

"I can see why you succeeded when you pitched this form of corporate giving to executives. You make a pretty compelling case."

"Well, it's true that I told this to executives and other stakeholders. But the value of serving others extends to everyone. You know, we engaged the people we helped in the helping, too. That was perhaps the most empowering way we helped them. To help them, help us, help them—that was the most beautiful aspect, to me."

In addition to Glen's service work, he had gone on retreats in various parts of the world, often hosted by tribal communities. He said those experiences helped reinforce his sense of humility and his commitment to environmental causes. So, in quite a number of ways, Glen was a deeply spiritual and evolved guy.

Identifying the Sources of the Fears

In a sense, Glen's evolved state created a problem for us. He was so well put together that it was difficult to identify what kind of help he was seeking from me. Also, he wasn't clear about articulating it. That's not unusual in psychotherapy. Clients and I often use the first few sessions to define the treatment goals.

One day, during our process of clarifying the focus of our work, I remarked, "You know, Glen, in our first session, you told me you came to see me because your surgeon recommended it. You said you agreed it's probably a good idea to explore whether there are any issues that a cosmetic procedure might bring to the surface. I don't want you to feel like you have to have an answer, but I wonder: we've met two times. At this point, are you thinking of some ways I might help you?"

Glen shifted in the armchair and looked out the window. He sat, pensive, and then said, "I feel somewhat embarrassed. The answer is I just don't want to feel so concerned about my appearance. This may sound arrogant, but I feel like it's beneath me. It feels so shallow and weak, and yet the truth is I do feel concerned. And I know my concerns are warranted. I know my industry. I've seen six executives leave in the past ten years. And I heard the talk. I know how they were perceived. They were thought to be out of touch."

"You don't sound shallow or weak to me, Glen. And I don't know your business the way you do, but I know how often people talk about the reality of ageism. So, we could do some work focused on coping with that reality. There's something else that's important for any cosmetic patient to evaluate. And that is, how confident are you that this service can provide the benefits you seek?"

"I'm pretty confident," he replied. "I've been living in fear. The aging thing has felt like a ticking time bomb. This feels like a way to slow that progression. I just don't want the fear anymore. I'm over it. I've been losing sleep over this whole issue for months. Maybe years."

"It sounds like this is something you've thought about a lot."

"Oh, you have no idea," he said. "It's probably been two to three years that I've been more intensely focused on it. I really think this is a way to eliminate the age issue—for now."

Glen wanted a cosmetic procedure that would be limited in scope. He found a renowned oculofacial plastic surgeon who specialized in an upper eyelid procedure. Glen met with that doctor, who confirmed he was a good candidate for it.

Perceived risks and benefits of any surgical procedure are always important to explore with a prospective patient. In terms of the risks, Glen had a lot of confidence in his surgeon. That's always helpful. Many patients need help recognizing that confidence in the surgeon is more the result of a conscious decision than of finding objective facts. Ultimately, the patient needs to *decide* to believe in their surgeon. Fortunately for Glen, he did believe in his surgeon and seemed to counterbalance that confidence with a healthy awareness that there is always some risk in a surgical procedure.

Glen's challenges arose when we turned to the subject of the benefits he sought from the procedure. I observed that when Glen spoke of these benefits, his discussion extended beyond his professional life. This surprised me. I also felt curious because there was a different quality I saw in Glen when he spoke about his hopes for the procedure. I saw a level of desperation and urgency that I didn't understand. It seemed out of place in him.

When I noticed this, I said, "Glen, I understand your motives for having the procedure. And your aesthetic goals for the procedure sound realistic. You've said you also feel confident about that. And yet your sleep is still disturbed. And I sense there's an intense fear within you when you consider the prospect of the procedure failing. Is that an accurate description of what you're experiencing?"

Glen sat quietly. He glanced at the hills, as he often did when he was deep in thought. Then he said, with equal parts conviction and puzzlement, "I feel like I need to get this done. To be honest, I'm still not sure why it feels so urgent. But it does. And yes, the fear is intense. It's less than it was, but it's still intense."

Figure/Ground: When Fears Aren't What They Appear to Be

Glen's sense of foreboding seemed to involve more than concern over his continued professional viability. I believed Glen when he described his company's youth-centric culture, but I wasn't convinced that was the real issue. I suspected that Glen's concerns about aging out of his workplace might have been covering up something deeper, related to what psychologists refer to as existential and life-stage development issues.

Existential issues that arise in psychotherapy generally involve the client's struggle with the value and meaning of their existence. Life-stage development issues refer to the stages of development we all pass through, throughout our lives. Theorists who have written about the stages of life often identify certain tasks or challenges that people confront at different stages. These theories contend that, every seven to twelve years, depending on the theory, we reevaluate our lives, consciously or unconsciously. During those reevaluation periods, we assess the choices we have made and the current direction of our lives. Sometimes these periods prompt individuals to change course by altering some major past decisions such as one's spouse, career, or place of residency.

The actual issues contributing to Glen's struggle crystallized during one session when he discussed his childhood. "My mom and dad had that kind of old-fashioned devotion to each other. Each was the other's biggest fan. My mom ran a tight ship. Dinner was on the table at six sharp every night. My sister and I had to have our hands and nails clean. Mom would check them. Mom was quiet, but she was a strong Irish Catholic woman. She took pride in the home she made, and in the term 'homemaker.' She used to say, 'houses are built, homes are made'."

Glen spoke of his mother lovingly and respectfully. When the subject turned to his father, Glen became much more animated and full of emotion. "My dad was a force. His personality filled the room. He was the quintessential, belly-laughing, back-slapping salesman. Everybody loved my dad. He was real active in the Knights of Columbus charitable organization, and that kept him busy when he wasn't working. There was always a meeting, a fundraiser, or a service event. And my mom was so devoted. She enjoyed him but she liked alone time. She was happy to stay at home and take care of my sister and me and the house. My parents made a great team." Saying this activated strong emotions in Glen.

"Can you stay with that emotion, Glen? Tell me about what you're feeling."

"I'm thinking about my dad. I miss him. He died in 1986, but I lost him around six years before that." Glen paused and wiped his eyes with a tissue. He took some breaths to help him tamp down his tears. Later in his treatment, we examined his habit of cutting off feelings of sadness before taking the opportunity to explore them. Glen continued, "I must have been about thirty-five. I was working in the city, and my mom started calling me at work. She had never done that. She would ask me questions about my dad's behavior, and she'd tell me not to mention it to anyone. By the time she began calling me, she had been seeing symptoms for months. My sister and I hadn't noticed, and my mother hadn't told us because she knew he didn't want anyone to know."

"He had early onset Alzheimer's?" I asked.

"Yeah, that's what it was. He started forgetting things, like how to do things. He'd get lost driving back from client visits. Much later, Mom told us there were times he'd show up in the middle of the night or the next morning. She knew he wasn't having an affair." Glen paused, took a tissue, and breathed a few times to tamp down his sadness.

"When I think of the nights she spent alone, wondering and worrying about him, and him out there alone and lost. I still think back about it and wonder how many times it happened. And how many angels are out there who he cajoled into pointing him in the right direction. It makes me very sad to think about all of that. I'm sad that I couldn't help them." Glen wiped his eyes and took several more breaths in and out.

"Take your time. See if you can allow yourself to stay with the emotions."

Glen continued, "I'm okay. It's just that he was always so vibrant and happy, and he became so irritable and so easily frustrated. He began to stay at home more often, probably because he was afraid of getting lost. For a long while, he wouldn't go to a doctor, and Mom felt his wishes should be respected. My sister and I disagreed, but we knew my mom wasn't going to budge. And then it all hit the fan. He was driving home from a client visit and crashed the car. He didn't get hurt, but that led to the diagnosis. It was the beginning of a very fast decline. The company didn't know what to do about it. People wanted to help, but nobody knew what to do back then. This was around 1980. He stopped working within a year and he died within six years."

"That's very sad, Glen. I'm sorry."

After Glen's description of his father's final years, Glen's struggle, and the focus of our work together, became clearer. His thoughts of his own aging process were occurring within the context of his father's misfortune. The sense of urgency he felt about the cosmetic work was real, but it covered a deeper, more profound fear. Glen was struggling with the reality that misfortune and particularly health-related issues can strike at any time, and are more likely to surface as we age. The real issue Glen was confronting was his fear that his father's fate would ultimately be his own fate.

Glen's aging issues caused him to consider the arc of his career. Thinking of that led Glen to think about the arc of his entire life. Glen was concerned he might be pushed out of the firm, but the more we discussed that situation, the more it became clear that his position was secure. That fear was masking a more poignant struggle with his own mortality and with the value and meaning of the life he had led.

Glen felt so fearful that he might develop Alzheimer's disease that he had always avoided speaking about it with anyone, including doctors. He believed he could undergo testing to determine his susceptibility, but he chose not to do that because he feared he couldn't cope with an Alzheimer's diagnosis. As he approached the age when his father was diagnosed, he became more and more focused on any symptom of decline or aging.

In psychotherapy, sometimes issues emerge that neither the therapist nor the client saw coming. Glen entered psychotherapy thinking he needed to have a healthy mindset regarding the cosmetic changes. In the end, Glen's psychotherapy had little to do with the cosmetic procedure. Those concerns fell away once we uncovered the true source of his difficulties.

Glen's surgical procedure went well. He was happy with the outcome. His psychotherapy explored his values and the ways they influenced the major decisions he had made in his life. We also devoted a lot of attention to his tendency, within his own mind, to diminish his achievements. No amount of service felt like it was enough for Glen. He felt blessed, which was healthy, but he used that awareness to punish himself.

Glen benefited from various meditations. Three to four times each week, he did Tonglen meditations. He found those to be the most effective type of meditation in his pursuit of feeling more closely connected to a sense of gratitude. And he did three to four loving kindness meditations per week in order to practice being kinder toward himself. He also decided to plan another service mission in a different part of the world.

Fears about the Surgery Experience: Anesthesia

Let's now examine one of the most feared issues associated with a surgical procedure: the anesthetic. It's common for patients to have difficulty trusting the safety of anesthesia. Some patients fear a disabling or deadly anesthetic dosage error could occur. Others worry that the anesthetic will stop working during the procedure, causing them to suddenly become conscious and able to feel pain.

I've found it helpful to advise patients to speak directly with the anesthesiologist. Many patients don't realize that anesthesiologists are medical doctors and specialists, just like surgeons. One anesthesiologist described his role this way: "Surgeons are like real good mechanics. The surgeon knows exactly what needs to be fixed and how to fix it, like a mechanic working on a car. The anesthesiologist makes sure the car will start up again once the surgeon fixes it." The anesthesiologist monitors not only the anesthetic drugs, but also the person's respiration and heart-related functions, fluid administration, and everything else required to maintain the patient's health throughout the surgical procedure. These measures also play a central role in the patient's recovery.

So, the anesthesiologist is a fully-licensed, well-trained, and experienced specialist physician who is actively involved throughout the surgical procedure. Although anesthesia accidents do happen, they are rare, particularly when an anesthesiologist is administering the anesthesia.

When you seek reassurance from the anesthesiologist, it helps to have clear, concise questions. Over the years, clients have raised various concerns with me. I compiled the following list of questions, based on these concerns.

Questions to Ask the Anesthesiologist:

1. What medications do you intend to use?

2. How long should I expect to be unconscious?

3. What happens if the anesthetic does not make me unconscious?

4. Is it possible the anesthetic could render me unable to speak, but leave me conscious and feeling pain?

5. Do patients ever wake up in the middle of the procedure?

6. Do patients ever die due to the anesthesia? Why? How common is that?

7. Why do people sometimes become brain-damaged due to a general anesthetic? Which patients are more at risk of that?

8. Who monitors the anesthetic during the surgery?

9. Am I at greater risk if the surgery is longer than a certain number of hours? If so, how many hours, why is there more risk, and how can I minimize it?

10. Does my weight, or do any of my other health characteristics, make me a more difficult person to anesthetize?

11. Should I stop using alcohol, marijuana, or other substances? How long before the procedure must I stop?

12. What other information can you provide that will help ease my anxiety?

It's helpful to note that the above discussion assumes a board-certified anesthesiologist will administer the anesthesia. While this is often the case, it is not always so. Sometimes a nurse anesthetist or the physician performing the procedure administers the anesthesia. When that is the case, I recommend that the patient ask the surgeon the above questions and gain the surgeon's reassurance that the procedure will be safe. Patients in this situation may want to consult an independent anesthesiologist as well.

Managing Fear During Recovery: Monitoring Healing

For many patients, the struggle with fears does not end once the surgery is over. The ultimate outcome of a surgical cosmetic service normally takes months to reveal itself. Our bodies need time to heal. Patients often continue to struggle with their fears even if there were no complications.

For a variety of reasons, it can be difficult for some patients to manage their post-procedural anxiety. One reason is surgeons typically need their patients to monitor healing. For example, most surgical procedures cause temporary swelling. A gradual reduction in swelling is a sign of normal healing, and someone needs to monitor the swelling to confirm the healing process is proceeding normally. Also, bandages need to be changed and sutures might need to be observed and sometimes cleaned. Some complications, such as infections, need to be addressed right away. The physician typically informs the patient of what will be needed during the recovery period and of any symptoms that should raise concerns.

For some patients, wound monitoring is very stressful. I've heard many patients report feeling the need for more guidance than their surgeon provided for this monitoring. Patients have sometimes said they feel unable to recognize such things as when a bruise is changing color or when swelling is decreasing. Sometimes their anxiety causes them to doubt their observations.

Another issue that can compromise a patient's assessment of their own healing is their discomfort. Postoperative monitoring can be difficult for a patient distracted by physical and/or emotional pain. Emotional pain can be experienced in many ways. Two examples are fear or disgust at the sight of the wound. These difficulties can cause some patients to be too consumed with emotions to arrive at an objective assessment of their wound.

It's unfortunately all too common for fears to detract from a patient's ability to monitor healing. Sophocles is credited with saying, "To him who is in fear, everything rustles." Indeed, people who struggle with anxiety tend to flood themselves with fears. One way they do this is by actively finding things to worry about. The cause of this behavior and the ways it can be interrupted and conquered will be described in Chapter 8. For our present purposes, it's important to recognize that anxiety threatens the patient's ability to provide their surgeon with accurate post-op progress reports.

Problems in monitoring reveal themselves in a number of ways. For instance, high anxiety causes a patient to be overly vigilant. This can lead them to describe the wound site inaccurately, implying the presence of complications that don't actually exist. This often happens when the patient monitors too frequently, a common problem with patients who have anxious tendencies. Other patients are on the other end of the monitoring continuum, feeling so fearful of looking at the wounds that they are unable to monitor their progress at all, placing themselves at risk of being totally unaware of a serious complication.

I was caught by surprise when I first ran across this issue. I was treating a very powerful person in the entertainment business. This person was fully aware of their anxious tendencies, and they wisely arranged to have one of their personal assistants present to monitor post-op healing. I thought this would avert any monitoring issues. It didn't. After the procedure, the patient was so anxious about the outcome that they decided they didn't want to be seen by anyone, even their assistant. So, they prevented their assistant from looking at the wounds.

I've seen this happen more than once. Very powerful people are accustomed to being surrounded by people who do whatever they say. During the post-op period, the person monitoring the wound must be permitted to do their job. I've learned that it's important to talk frankly with these clients and include their human monitors in some of the discussions. The patient and the monitor need to have an explicit agreement, prior to the procedure, that the monitor will have the final say regarding any issue connected to the monitoring task. Before the procedure, patients need to have a postsurgical plan that addresses these and any other issues that might prevent the patient from engaging in healthy healing behaviors.

Coping Tool: Managing Postoperative Anxiety

It's scary to undergo a cosmetic procedure. Both the patient and the physician have an interest in the patient managing their anxiety effectively. Throughout this book there are psychological practices and exercises that can help you train your brain to improve your resiliency. The following general practices are a good place to start in the process of preparing to skillfully manage postoperative anxiety:

Managing Post-operative Anxiety

1. Anxious patients should see a psychologist prior to the procedure in order to develop anxiety management skills.

2. Before the procedure, ask the surgeon to describe, in great detail, types of post-op observations that should raise concerns.

3. Adhere completely to the healing practices the surgeon provides.

4. Monitor your progress carefully enough to catch problems, but not so much as to go overboard with the monitoring.

5. Have a direct contact number for the surgeon's office for the days after the procedure, to ask questions or express concerns regarding the healing process.

6. Hire a nurse who has experience with healing from these procedures to visit your home and assist your monitoring and cleaning of your wounds. Physicians often have experienced nurses available for this purpose. This can be very reassuring, especially during the initial days after the procedure.

7. Some patients should not self-monitor. For some, looking into the mirror soon after the surgical procedure can provoke too much anxiety. Anxious people tend to be impatient, wanting to see positive results too soon. For these patients, it's best to have another person monitor their healing.

8. Bring a relative or friend to pre-surgical appointments. Have that person assist you during your healing. Encourage that person to play an active part in meetings with your surgeon, so that you have an ally who knows what must be done to facilitate your healing.

Should YOU Self-Monitor? The MIRROR Test

The benefits of psychotherapy notwithstanding, not all patients should self-monitor their postoperative healing. There are many ways anxiety can be a debilitating condition. For cosmetic patients, severe anxiety can threaten a patient's ability to safely and effectively self-monitor. The MIRROR Test is a tool that can help you assess the likelihood that self-monitoring might be overly difficult for you. MIRROR is an acronym derived from the statement *"Man, I Really, Really Often Recoil."* Like other screening tools in this book, The Mirror Test is not intended to tell you what you can and cannot do. Instead, it is a simple tool that you can use to explore the risks and benefits of self-monitoring.

To take the MIRROR Test, simply answer the following seven statements. For each, decide whether the statement describes you or not. Answer yes or no for each question.

1. I regularly take medication for anxiety, depression, bipolar symptoms (including "mood stabilizer" medications), or a psychotic condition.

2. On at least three days each week, I rely on non-prescription substances (such as marijuana) for relaxation.

3. I have experienced panic attacks or very high levels of anxiety.

4. I have undergone surgical procedures before, and experienced high anxiety during the healing process.

5. I feel very nervous about this procedure.

6. Positive results from this procedure will significantly improve my personal life and/or my professional life.

7. I am often troubled by thoughts of worst-case scenarios.

Scoring. If you answered "yes" to three or more items, self-monitoring will likely *not* be your most prudent choice. Find a medical professional or a trusted, levelheaded family member or friend to monitor your healing for you. At the very least, gain the support of a second or third person to monitor with you if you insist on self-monitoring.

If you answered "yes" to two items, the decision to self-monitor should be made only after carefully considering the risks. Ideally, you should have a medical professional, friend, or family member available to assist you in monitoring your healing progress.

If you answered "yes" to only one of the items, you will probably be able to self-monitor, but you will still benefit from having the support of a friend or family member.

If you answered "no" to all items, there is likely no reason to avoid postsurgical self-monitoring. But remember: everyone benefits from having the support of others, so you might still want to consider having someone available to help you out.

Coping Methods if You Choose Not to Self-Monitor

If, after assessing your situation, you have decided not to self-monitor, the next thing you should do is congratulate yourself. It takes courage to decide to allow others to support your healing. Being so self-aware is truly a strength worth celebrating. By making this decision, you are prioritizing self-care. That quality alone makes your healthy recovery more likely.

Now you need to make some plans that will ensure your healing is monitored in a way that you can trust. Below are several methods to help you accomplish that.

Coping Methods

1. Have people in your physician's office monitor your progress. Your physician's team offers the benefit of direct observation by trained individuals who can alert the physician if necessary. This option does have a few disadvantages. First, this method can be costly. Second, you may prefer not to leave home often, particularly in the days following the procedure. Finally, your physician might advise against this in favor of a method that permits more rest during your recovery.

2. If permitted by your doctor, use an alternative to office visits, like Zoom, Doxy, or another HIPAA-compliant videoconferencing tool. If you choose this method, be sure to conduct a dry run with the doctor's office prior to the procedure.

3. Have a friend or relative do the monitoring. The individual should be able to both monitor progress and assist you in managing your anxiety. Anxious patients often place high demands on the people assisting them. It's a good idea for both the monitor and the patient to be mindful of that prior to the procedure.

Future Fears: Losing Muscular Functionality

One concern I often hear surrounding cosmetic surgical work involves the fear that the physician will make a mistake, causing impairment in the use of muscles, such as those in the face. This fear is especially common for actors or models.

As with any fear, it's best to begin by carefully assessing its accuracy. You can do this by searching for information. The first source is your surgeon, but you will also want to consult other sources, including reputable web-based sources and even other surgeons. This fear provides another example of the value of choosing a surgeon with specialized expertise and experience in the particular procedure you seek. It's important to assess this concern with your surgeon with direct questions. For example, you might ask any of the following questions:

Questions About Losing Muscular Function

1. Is it possible to lose muscular functionality in the area where you will perform the procedure?

2. Why would this complication happen?

3. If it were to happen, how widespread could it be?

4. How do you prevent this?

5. Have you had patients experience this complication?

6. On a scale of 1–100, with 0 being no chance and 100 being a certainty, what is the likelihood that I will experience this complication?

7. How likely is it that such an outcome would be permanent?

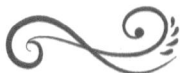

CHAPTER 8

Emotional and Physical Coping: What a Pain

You, yourself, as much as anybody in the entire universe, deserve your love and affection.

— **Buddha**

Knowing Pain

"Is it so unreasonable to want to know exactly what pain I'm going to endure? I just don't understand why that's such a sensitive question to ask a surgeon. Why couldn't he just answer it? It was like my surgeon had a panic attack just because I had questions."

When I met Elliot he was a forty-two-year-old commercial real estate developer. His wife of ten years was an attorney who specialized in medical malpractice. They had two sons, ages six and eight. He was preparing for a liposuction procedure and he was struggling. His experience will help us explore how our relationship with pain can become destructive. We will also examine the ways the surgeon-patient relationship can support a patient's process.

Wanting To Vent

Elliot's planned procedure was called 4D High-Def VASER liposuction. At that time, it was a relatively new form of liposuction. VASER liposuction removes fat by a different method than traditional liposuction. It aims to produce a sculpted physique. For our purposes, one of the other key differences is that the surgeon works on multiple areas of the body during one surgical procedure. Elliot's surgeon, we'll call him Dr. Hansen, referred Elliot to me because he thought Elliot seemed too anxious about the procedure.

In replying to Elliot's rhetorical questions about pain, I said, "I'm glad you asked me those questions. From a psychological perspective, you're smart to want to feel informed about your procedure. Knowledge can help you manage your anxiety. Would you mind telling me more about your concerns and questions?"

Elliot replied, "First, this is a complex procedure. Hansen will work on several areas during the same operation: my chest, stomach, back, and arms. That's a big deal. It's a lot to do in one procedure, so I'd like to know more about the risks. Also, he insists on using general anesthetic. That's another issue I can accept, but I'm not thrilled about it. Do you know how many lawsuits my wife has brought on behalf of patients whose doctors screwed up the anesthesia?"

"Based on your experience through your wife's work, I can see why that would be pretty scary," I said. "So, the anesthesia is one of your concerns?"

"Of course it is. It's general anesthesia! Do you know how dangerous general anesthesia is? Do you know how many people are injured by bad anesthesia? I'll probably pay off both of my kids' four-year college tuition bills with the money my wife earned off anesthesia errors."

Elliot's comments presented an opportunity for me to get a sense of his openness to examining his anxiety. "As it happens," I said, "I do know something about anesthesia risk. It's common for patients to talk with me about it, so I've learned more about it over the years. Before we talk about it, it'll help me to ask a preliminary question. Do you have ideas about how your work with me might help you deal with the fear of an error involving anesthesia?

"I guess I just want somewhere to vent," Elliot replied. "I majored in psych at UCLA. I believe in it. I mean, it's good to vent. It helps. I don't expect you to work miracles. I know that you can't take away the risk."

"I'm glad you're open to using our time to vent your feelings and thoughts. I agree—venting can be helpful. And of course, you're right that I can't take away the risk, but there's actually a lot more we can do in addition to giving you a place to vent. Do you remember I said the cognitive part of our work focuses on thinking accurately?"

"Yes, I remember that," Elliot said.

"Great. Well, our work together can help you get in the habit of checking your accuracy, such as when you think about risks. A commitment to accuracy, and then practicing maintaining it, is likely to be much more helpful than venting alone would be."

"Well, I can promise you that I'm accurate about anesthesia risk. I've seen enough of my wife's cases to know that anesthesia is very risky."

"Yes, it can be risky. And I know there have been accidents. Let's delve deeper into the cognitive work for a minute. Do you remember way back in your Intro to Psychology course, you learned about the availability heuristic?"

"You've got to be kidding. Do you realize that was about nineteen years and twenty-six pounds of weed ago?" We laughed, and Elliot continued, "No, I definitely do not remember that. I'm all ears."

"Okay, well, it's pretty simple," I said. "The availability heuristic refers to the tendency we have to think that something familiar to us is more common than it actually is. It seems common because we happen to see a bunch of it. A heuristic is like a mental shortcut. So, the availability heuristic would suggest that your preexisting knowledge of your wife's medical malpractice cases might cause you to think medical malpractice is more common than it actually is."

"Well, I can promise you," Elliot replied, "people die from anesthesia."

"For sure. I know that has happened. And it doesn't do us any good to try to deny that. What do you think the alternative to denial would be?"

"Honestly, aside from talking about it, I don't know."

"What you said is actually the core of the answer—we talk about it. But we need to talk in a particular way. We need to be analytical and accurate. We need to use the cognitive work to reduce the anxiety. So, for instance, just because an anesthesia error could be very dangerous, that doesn't mean it's likely. We use our conversations to check the accuracy of the thoughts that are fueling our fears."

"But how do you know it's not likely? Maybe it's very likely," Elliot said.

"That's right. So, we need to go find the answer. We need data. And this is why we sometimes do research as part of the psychotherapy. One way to deal with anxiety is to acquire information. So, before our next session, you have an assignment. Do some online research. Try to find out how often there are anesthesia errors in cosmetic interventions and bring it to your next session with me. Remember a few things. First, compare apples to apples. If your procedure will have an anesthesiologist present, your data should only refer to errors by anesthesiologists. Next, try to remember to bring the information plus the sources of the information. And finally, remember it's best to get info from multiple sources."

At our next session, Elliot brought information indicating that, in fact, anesthesia has become much safer over the past twenty years or so.

His research confirmed that anesthesiologists have many ways of monitoring patients during surgery. And new technology has led to new and more effective methods in recent decades, making it much less likely a patient will have a serious injury due to an anesthetic.

Worries Compounding Worries

"So, Elliot, now that you have confirmation that a serious anesthesia injury is very unlikely, have you noticed whether the intensity of your fear has changed?"

"Well, about that, yes," Elliot said. "But it didn't eliminate other fears. There are a lot of things that could go wrong, not just the anesthetic."

"Great. Let's talk about one of those. What concern do you want us to take up next?"

"Do you remember what I said about the nature of this kind of liposuction procedure?"

"I do," I replied. "I remember you mentioned you felt concerned about the riskiness of Hansen operating on several areas during the same operation. Do you want to focus on that today?"

"Sure."

"Great. Did you ask Hansen about that when you met with him?"

"Sure did."

"Good! And what did he say about it?"

"He said very little, that's what he said. He was vague. He just gave me a prepared answer. You know, this is what he does all the time, there's nothing to worry about. Blah, blah, blah. There was no substance. His answer was essentially 'trust me'."

"So, you didn't feel like he satisfied your concerns."

"No way. It was all fluff. And he still hasn't answered my questions about the pain. I just don't know what kind of pain to expect. When I asked Hansen, he said, 'You'll need to take it easy for the first few days, but then it should start getting better,' or something vague like that. I want more details. I asked him what will hurt the most, and he couldn't say. He just said every patient is different, but he'll give me pain medicine."

"Are you saying you don't believe him that patients differ in those respects?" I asked.

"I'm just saying I know he doesn't have a crystal ball, but I don't believe he can't tell me more. I mean, will the back hurt most or will the chest? Or will I just hurt all over? Am I not going to be able to move at all because of the pain? And if that's the case, how much painkiller will I need? And how will I avoid becoming addicted? Also, I get sick from pills. I hate medications. What if I vomit and the painkiller doesn't take effect? I'm afraid the pain might be unbearable. There's so much uncertainty, and he has not provided much relief at all."

Elliot identified multiple sources of fear. It was clear we would need to discuss pain management, coping with the reality of risk in a complex procedure, and his perception that his doctor wasn't entirely invested in his procedure. We also needed to discuss Elliot's perception that his doctor was unable to communicate with Elliot in a way that was reassuring. As we will discuss in Chapter 11, if the patient has found the right doctor, the discussions with that doctor will leave the patient feeling relieved and reassured.

Larger than any of those specific issues was a much broader issue: Elliot's habitual tendency to maintain a state of anxiety within himself. We weren't ready to tackle that yet, but to help him effectively, we would need to address it eventually.

Elliot, like so many people who struggle with anxiety, had a tendency to jump from one source of anxiety to another without stopping to identify coping tools for any of them. The anxiety becomes like a giant snowball rolling down a steep hill and getting larger and larger.

The snowball effect happens because people who struggle with anxiety tend to ignore their successes in conquering sources of anxiety. This causes them to preserve the sense of overwhelm. They feel as though they have too many things on their plate—too many sources of anxiety—to manage any of them.

During a psychotherapy session, I often stop the client and urge them to notice that we solved one of the issues they mentioned. So, something was removed from their plate. I draw their attention to that achievement. We need to celebrate that the plate's contents are fewer and also the idea that we are able to eliminate things from the plate.

A fundamental aspect of anxiety treatment is confidence building. The client needs to see that by diminishing their own successes they overlook their ability to help themselves, which perpetuates their anxiousness. The sense of helplessness and inadequacy reinforces the anxious state.

This kind of dynamic can even occur in a person like Elliot, who is a successful, smart guy. A lot of people do a much better job appearing calm than feeling calm. Elliot was definitely one of those people. It was only the multitude of questions that led Elliot's surgeon to recognize the anxiety issue.

In the ten weeks leading up to Elliot's procedure, we devoted a lot of focus to helping him see his tendency to flood himself with fears. He reported that he used a mindfulness meditation daily to work on creating more space in his mind. The objective was for Elliot to acquire the skill of slowing down his tendency to react to every thought.

Using Our Mindset to Cope with Physical Pain

Not surprisingly, surgical patients often fear painful recoveries. Unfortunately, most cosmetic procedures do involve some postprocedural physical discomfort. It's surprising, though, how often patients report that the discomfort was not only tolerable but was much briefer and much less unpleasant than they expected.

We know that patients who cope most effectively with pain interpret their pain in healthy ways. Clients are often surprised to hear that there are healthy ways to experience pain. This is one way psychotherapy can be helpful to someone in pain.

A growing body of research indicates that our thoughts have influence over our pain tolerance. It turns out we can actually make our pain feel worse by how we think about it. Sit with that idea for a moment. The way you *think* can actually cause you to *feel* more or less pain. That's a pretty powerful idea. Our job in psychotherapy is to use that powerful idea to help the client feel empowered.

All of this does not mean pain is a mere product of our imaginations. Pain and discomfort are very real, but there are psychological methods that can help us manage the discomfort in ways that actually diminish our perception of its intensity.

For the cosmetic patient, there are a number of benefits to improved pain management. The first and most obvious benefit is that we have a more enjoyable recovery if we feel like our pain has been adequately managed. Better pain management tends to help us maintain a more hopeful mood and mindset. The more hopeful your mood, the more likely you'll engage in healthy behaviors like eating healing foods, sleeping enough, and caring for your body in the ways your doctor advised.

Another benefit of effective pain management is that people who manage their discomfort tend to require less assistance from others. Being more independent engenders a sense of empowerment, which is also beneficial to healing. There's no doubt about it: effective pain management serves everyone's interests.

I've never known a surgical patient who wasn't prescribed pain medication. As a psychologist, I would never tell a patient to take or to reject a medication. I do, however, actively encourage my clients to integrate these nonpharmacologic methods of pain management. One reason is that the non-drug methods often help, sometimes very much. Another reason I do this is that pharmacologic pain management can be ineffective or even counterproductive. This is why psychological treatment is now generally recognized as an excellent alternative or adjunctive treatment to pharmacologic pain management. The final reason I give to clients for adding non-drug pain management to their regimen is "it couldn't hurt."

For a patient like Elliot, psychological pain management was particularly important. Dr. Hansen was right: Elliot struggled too much with his fear of physical discomfort. So, one of the goals Elliot and I set in the initial sessions was for him to enhance his ability to use coping skills to better manage pain.

At the outset, Elliot and I needed to examine his thoughts and feelings about pain.

In one of our early sessions, I suggested, "I think we should talk about the psychology of pain tolerance."

Elliot immediately attempted to lighten the mood. Leaning forward and grabbing the caffe latte he brought into the session, he said, before taking a swig, "You mean you want to discuss how I can wish my pain away? I'm willing, but, to be honest, Doc, I don't think I'll succeed." Elliot was joking, but he was also letting me know that he wanted me to respect not only his pain but also his fear of it.

I decided to do that with humor. "Are you ready to hear something you're gonna think is even more crazy than wishing your pain away?"

"Are you kidding?" Elliot replied, playing along. "I'd love to hear that!"

"Okay, here goes. What may sound even more crazy is that, actually, in psychotherapy for pain management, not only do we *not* try to wish the pain away, but we actually do the opposite. We invite our pain to come closer. We practice intentionally coexisting with our pain. Some people even describe it as befriending our pain."

Elliot broke into a genuine laugh, which made me laugh, too. As a meditation convert, I totally related to his reaction. He took another sip of his coffee, sat back, and crossed one leg over the other. "Listen, I like you. Don't take this to be disrespectful, but that sounds like the typical psychobabble that I was afraid I'd run into in a psychotherapy office. Pain is pain. You can quote me on that, by the way. Pain is pain. If pain were enjoyable, they wouldn't have called it pain."

"I hear you. And don't worry about being disrespectful. I didn't and won't take anything you say personally. In fact, your directness is really helpful to our work."

I proceeded to explain the following to Elliot: "One goal of psychological pain management is accurate thinking. The research in this area is unequivocal. We can actually intensify our pain by treating it as though it's unacceptable or intolerable. Some people are so uncomfortable with even the idea of pain that they focus all their energy on avoiding it. We actually increase our pain by refusing to coexist with it."

"I guess I can understand that concept, but I don't really know what to do with it. I mean, I can't picture myself just sitting and enjoying pain. I can't even picture what sitting with my pain would look like."

"That's a helpful reaction," I said, "because I've told you that this work isn't about lying to yourself. So, it makes sense that something we know to be unpleasant, like pain, would not be something we would enjoy being with. The first answer is, the objective is not to enjoy the pain, exactly. You direct your efforts simply at achieving acceptance of it, peaceful coexistence with it. You don't need to become best friends with pain, but you also don't want to think of your pain as an enemy you must vanquish. That's what intensifies the discomfort."

"So, first of all, I heard the 'exactly.' You said that I'm not going to try to enjoy the pain exactly, which means I'll enjoy it somewhat, which still sounds ridiculous to me. But I'll set that aside and just ask from a thoughts perspective, how do I not want my pain to go away?" Elliot asked.

"There are different methods. One is to notice the pain but with a curious mindset. Imagine you're a scientist writing a magazine article titled 'Exactly What My Pain Feels Like.' Or imagine you have a very curious Martian friend, who can understand earthling words but cannot feel pain and so has no idea what pain is. The Martian wants you to describe it very precisely. Either imaginary task would require you to distinguish among the sensations. That process helps you to detach somewhat from the discomfort. You could use either of these methods to document in writing each component of the pain: burning, pulsing, itching, stinging, tickling, cooling, pulling, pressing, and so on. You might choose to compare the feelings to something you've felt before. This activity can take your mind away from the reactive behavior we're used to of just rejecting the pain. Do you want to hear about another method?"

"Sure," Elliot replied.

"Another way of embracing pain is essentially by focusing on gratitude. You can make a conscious effort to be aware of the way pain serves your body. Pain sensations can be thought of as your body's way of telling you there's healing happening. In this way, discomfort can be experienced as evidence that your body is fighting on your behalf. If you think of discomfort that way, you can justify befriending it, rather than considering it to be a weapon wielded against you by an enemy."

"I can't believe I'm about to say this, but I get that. It makes sense," Elliot replied.

"Great. So, the practice of monitoring our pain becomes a kind of mindfulness practice. This is why meditation, which is about practicing coexisting with everything within and outside of ourselves, is such a powerful tool, and so relevant to pain management. If you're willing, I have a mindfulness meditation I can give you that encourages you to sit in peace, so to speak, with your discomfort, to get to know it. Then the practice can help you see the discomfort evolve over time. I don't want to lie to you, Elliott, mindfulness meditation is difficult, but many people have found it helpful, particularly if used repeatedly."

"I'm not thinking it sounds easy," Elliot said. "I'm thinking it sounds easier to say than to do."

"There's no question that's true. It's very difficult. All meditation requires practice because it's counterintuitive. Our instincts tell us to push pain away and pull pleasure to ourselves. But that isn't self-care. Coexisting with both pain and pleasure is self-care because both exist. Acceptance of both represents acceptance of our reality. One final benefit to bear in mind, Elliot, is effective pain management maximizes your healing because it helps you to monitor your healing and respond accurately to your condition."

I explained that coexisting with pain can also be achieved through distraction. Distractions can give us a break from some or all of the pain and are therefore a powerful tool in pain management. This is another benefit of having a supportive person spend time with you during your recovery.

"Well, of course distractions are helpful," Elliot said, "but that's just the point. There's no escape from the pain. We feel pain all the time when we are in pain."

"I get what you're saying," I said. "The thing is, and I know this will sound harsh, but you have to accept some responsibility for choosing that way of thinking about pain. The undeniable fact is that some people do cope with pain better than other people. And we know that the reason is they react differently to the pain. So, for instance, they choose to distract themselves with things to do when they are experiencing pain. They take a walk, bake a cake, make Jell-O, walk the dog, play with the cat, do something artistic, clean something, watch a favorite show—they do anything that, even partially, takes them away from focusing exclusively on the pain. Now, ignoring the pain might be very difficult. That's true. But you and I both know it's also true that you ultimately have the power to undermine the power of any distraction. If you're baking a cake and aren't really engaged in the activity, and are focusing constantly on the pain, you'll be less likely to benefit from the distraction. Using your mind in these ways requires a conscious and intentional commitment."

Using Mindfulness Meditation to Cope with Physical Pain

The descriptions of alternative ways of thinking about pain, and of experiencing pain, seemed to help Elliot. I find that most clients share his reactions, including the sort of brightening in his face that I saw after he heard there are ways of coping. He seemed more hopeful but remained appropriately skeptical. His observations were insightful. He asked a lot of questions and they were direct and rational.

"This sounds sensible," he said. "But something occurs to me. We do things well that we practice. So, one lingering question I have is: how do I practice this? I'm not in pain now. How can I learn to do this if I'm not in pain?"

"You're right. Practice prepares you for the real thing. One form of practice is meditation. You can do the Mindfulness Meditation for Pain even if you aren't in pain. You do it by focusing on any sensation: an itch, a hunger pang, dry eye, chapped lips, a cuticle that needs clipping, feeling cold or warm, and so on. The sensation can even be one that isn't annoying, like the feeling of the floor underneath your feet. The objective is to stop and focus on any sensation. Instead of scratching the itch, try to observe it. In other words, try to practice coexisting with the itch instead of removing it by scratching."

"So," Elliot said, "when I meditate, I'm never trying to remove certain thoughts or feelings? Even unhealthy ones?"

"Exactly," I said. "Instead of scratching the itch, you notice it, and you then focus on your breathing, to resist acting by instinct. You want to try to allow all elements of all sensations to enter your awareness. If you feel intolerant toward a sensation, or a thought, try to be aware of that, and curious about the part of you that feels that way. And, Elliot, above all else, try to remember to be patient with yourself. This is difficult. It should take time to develop this completely new response pattern."

I suggested Elliot begin regularly using the Mindfulness Meditation for Pain well in advance of his procedure. I gave him the formal instructions for this meditation that are provided at the end of this chapter. I want to briefly mention one coping method that I gave Elliot that is not in the instructions. This involves a method for helping yourself maintain focus during the meditation. You can count every inhalation until your attention wanes. When you notice your attention wane, note the number you reached. On the next inhalation, begin the count again. See how high you can get that count. Counting breaths can help you improve your ability to remain present and observe whatever physical sensations, thoughts, or emotions may enter your consciousness.

Addressing the Tendency to Worry

Elliot had lingering doubts about his surgeon. I felt a desire to address them, both for Elliot's sake and his surgeon's sake. I no longer practice law, but my training and experience in law made it difficult to ignore the specter of a malpractice lawsuit, given Elliot's wife's area of practice. My concern was not Dr. Hansen's skill level; it was the real damage that can be done if a patient doesn't trust the surgeon. The risk of noncompliance and other counterproductive patient behaviors led me to believe it would be best to address the issue with Elliot.

I was aware Elliot still viewed Dr. Hansen as dismissive and not very approachable. Elliot felt treated like just another patient or, worse yet, like an annoying patient. I encouraged Elliot to create another set of questions to bring to Dr. Hansen.

We constructed these questions together. He agreed to call Dr. Hansen's office and request a time to talk. Dr. Hansen created a special appointment, at the end of his day when he was usually not in the office, to meet with Elliot. I first learned all this from Dr. Hansen himself. I didn't know when or whether Elliot had followed through until I got a text message from Dr. Hansen, asking me to speak with him.

It turned out they met a few days after my session with Elliot. Minutes after Elliot left his office, Dr. Hansen texted me, asking for a brief phone conversation.

I agreed to talk with him, but I needed to take steps to protect Elliot's privacy. I didn't have permission from Elliot to talk with Dr. Hansen. This meant I couldn't share any information with Dr. Hansen about Elliot— even the fact that I knew Elliot.

When I answered my phone, Dr. Hansen began, "I sent a patient of mine to talk with you. I think I told you once that my wife is a psychologist, so I know you cannot confirm that you're seeing him, and I don't need you to do that. And I also don't want you to share any of his private information with me. So, I don't think you need a release to talk with me. Mainly I just want to tell you about my concerns. I know this is an unusual request, but can we try this?"

"Sure, we can," I replied. "Let me just tell you a couple things about how I handle these situations. As you said, without a release from a patient, I can't share any information at all. So, I can hear information from you, and I can comment on it, but my comments will be general and will use only information you provide me, as opposed to being based on any information I have about one of my patients."

"I understand. That's fine," Dr Hansen replied.

"Great. So, the final piece is that, if I am in fact treating your patient, I will probably need to tell the client that I spoke with you. I need to prioritize the relationship with my patients over relationships with other people. I wouldn't want the patient to think I was keeping a secret between me and you. Of course, I'd want to do it in a supportive way that wouldn't rupture your relationship with the patient."

"I don't have a problem with that, Alan," Dr. Hansen replied.

"Great. So, how can I help?"

"Of course, this is about Elliot. Alan, to be honest, I like the guy, but I've been considering asking him to find a different surgeon. I know you can't tell me anything, but I just wanted to tell you that his anxiety seems to be out of control. He almost seems manic."

"I'm glad you decided to talk with me. Can you describe the behaviors that caused you to feel concerned?"

"He's come to me twice with a sheet full of questions. I don't mind answering them, but it just seems like no answer satisfies him. I get a new sheet of questions every week, it seems. I've seen patients like him before. I'm concerned he's one of those people who's impossible to satisfy. My wife has warned me about patients like him. He's a squeaky wheel. I don't need to deal with a lawsuit. It's just not worth it."

"If he seems unsatisfied with your answers, I can see why you feel concerned. It may help you to know that I often encourage clients to construct a lot of questions for the surgeon, like the ones your patient brought to you. But I guess you're saying it was not the questions that bothered you as much as his dissatisfaction with your responses. Is that right?"

"I don't know. It's the questions, too, I suppose," Dr. Hansen said. "He just keeps coming back with questions. Endless questions. I've even met with him after normal business hours. Maybe you can tell me more about your process. I'm open to helping him cope with his fears, but I don't want to operate on someone who seems unstable. You know, the patient needs to adhere to a pretty involved healing regimen. His own anxiety could cause him to sue me because he could create a bad outcome by not complying with my instructions."

In a general way, I proceeded to describe the nature of the cognitive work that I do with patients. I explained that one of the best antidotes to anxiety is information, and that's why I encourage clients to ask a lot of questions. I then told him that meditation and mindfulness work do tend to help patients acquire more peace of mind prior to the procedure. Finally, there was something I wanted to tell Dr. Hansen about Elliot, but I knew I couldn't make it directly about Elliott. I did it this way:

"I think one more thing would be helpful for you to know: when someone is struggling with anxiety, it's common for them to jump from one source of anxiety to another. Often, before one issue gets addressed, the person focuses on another. I work with clients on that pretty actively. The goal-directed work we do in solution-focused psychotherapy really can help most high-functioning patients to curb that tendency. It occurs over a period of time and often in fits and starts. So that might give you some hope regarding the instability you're concerned about."

"That's very helpful," Dr. Hansen replied.

"I'm glad. One final thing might help. I remember when I was practicing law, I learned the maxim 'people sue people they don't like.' If that maxim remains true, it sounds to me like you're taking the right steps to avoid being sued. You said you made yourself available to talk with him, even after hours, you said you openly discussed his concerns and expectations, and you said you tried to put his mind at ease by giving him whatever information he sought."

"I really do want him to feel at ease on the day of the procedure," Dr. Hansen replied.

"If he is my client, I may be able to help. Of course, I would tell him that we spoke. I would also try to use the opportunity to help him see your good intentions. Your initiating the call and wanting to know how you could be supportive are exceptional qualities. I would hope I could help him to see that."

"I do appreciate that. Thanks very much."

When I met with Elliot, I described the broad outlines of my conversation with Dr. Hansen. As I'd hoped, Elliot was very happy to know that Dr. Hansen had called me. The call seemed to humanize Dr. Hansen in Elliot's eyes. Elliot was especially surprised to learn that Dr. Hansen had exhibited such a sincere interest in Elliot's emotional wellness. Elliot seemed to show Dr. Hansen a little more grace after he learned about his call to me.

I chose not to tell Elliot about Dr. Hansen's fear of being sued by him. I decided it wouldn't have been necessary or constructive to have shared that.

Dr. Hansen reported a distinct difference in Elliot, beginning in the weeks after his phone call. I believe that was directly the result of how Elliot felt about Dr. Hansen's efforts. Consistent with that, Elliot told me he felt more at ease with and trusting of Dr. Hansen.

During the remaining ten weeks prior to his procedure, Elliot acquired much more knowledge about what to expect. He also grew in his ability to accept the uncertainties. Meditation gradually helped him begin to develop the ability to quiet his mind. He did not evolve into an expert meditator in the months prior to his procedure, but he did enhance his ability to pause and lessen the intensity of his reactions to sources of anxiety.

Elliot's surgery went as expected. He reported that the meditations helped him remain calm in the hours prior to the procedure. After the procedure, Elliot reported to me that he planned to continue his meditation practice, though he would meditate less frequently than he did in the weeks prior to his procedure.

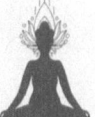

Exercise: Mindfulness Meditation for Coping with Pain

Reminder: a guided version of this meditation is located at DrAlanGoodwin.com

This meditation can be used to cope with pain, itching, or any unpleasant sensation.

1. Find a quiet, private place where you can practice staying present.

2. Assume a comfortable, relaxed position. You can sit or lie down, but it's best to remain awake. Choose an alert but relaxed position.

3. Take slow, deep breaths in and out. Breathe in a way that feels natural. If you can, exhale a bit longer than you inhale.

4. Notice whatever your five senses reveal. Take your time. As you breathe, identify any smells, sights, sounds, tastes, or feelings you perceive.

5. Continue the same breathing. Try to maintain your focus on your breaths. If your mind wanders, notice that you noticed it. That's good. You succeeded in being mindful. Acknowledge that your mind wandered and then gently remind yourself to return your focus to your breaths.

6. **Remember:** This is difficult. Try to embrace that.

7. As you breathe, notice any sensations. Take your time. Focus on any sensation with curiosity, like a research scientist would. Separate each sensation into its components. For instance, be curious about the location of it, the temperature, the nature of it, whether it is pulsing or constant, and any other feeling it brings. Is it sharp like a needle prick, or dull like an ache, or more like a cramp, or like an electrical shock? Notice the intensity. Is it changing? Does it come in waves? Try to be accurate.

8. Try to observe all aspects of each sensation, as you also focus on your breathing. If you notice yourself trying to push the sensation away, first notice that you succeeded in being mindful, then gently refocus on your breathing. Try to coexist with the sensation.

9. You may also notice your emotions. If you do, notice that you noticed. Good for you. You succeeded in being mindful. Acknowledge the emotion, then gently remind

yourself to return your focus to your breaths. (There is a different meditation that focuses on your emotions.)

10. Continue to focus on your breath and to breathe slowly and deeply. Continue to notice all sensations. Do this as long as you'd like.

11. When you decide to stop the meditation, devote some breaths to speaking mantras that praise yourself for doing the meditation. With each breath say a mantra that is brief, positive, accurate, and empowering. A few examples: *I am coping. I can cope. I am strong. I feel blessed. I am healing. Discomfort is temporary. I cope with pain. I coexist with pain.*

There is no minimum time for this exercise. Your practice session can be as brief as one minute, or as long as hours. Please remember to have patience with the process. Skills develop over time. It's best to begin to practice this exercise long before your planned procedure. In this way, you will begin your practice of focusing on body sensations when the context is an absence of pain. Remember that the objective of this exercise is not relaxation, it is presence. This meditation provides you practice remaining present with your body.

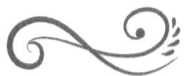

CHAPTER 9

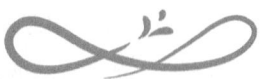

Coping with Knowing that You Don't Know

There are only two mistakes one can make along the road to truth: not going all the way, and not starting.

— Buddha

Coping with the Reality of Risk

We experience risk often. Anytime we do something without knowing what the outcome will be we are confronting the reality of risk. For cosmetic procedure patients, risk plays a particularly central role. Risk is inherent in these procedures, and the awareness of risk is prolonged because the outcome is unknown until some time after the procedure.

Tolerating uncertainty is very difficult for some people. When cosmetic patients become frustrated with the pace of the healing process, it sometimes leads to unhealthy behaviors. Those behaviors can not only delay proper healing; in extreme cases, the patient's behaviors can prevent proper healing. In this chapter, we will explore ways cosmetic surgery patients can enhance risk tolerance and reduce self-defeating behaviors to maximize the likelihood of achieving satisfying outcomes.

Risk Tolerance and Self-Confidence

Heather was a twenty-one-year-old nursing student when she began working with me in psychotherapy. When the world looked at Heather, it saw a friendly, unassuming, petite, and attractive young woman. Heather described herself in much less complimentary ways. She came to me for help with depressive symptoms. She had been dating David, a twenty-four-year-old MBA student, for about a year. She reported he would become upset with her fairly often. She felt confused by it and tried hard to rationalize his irritability. Heather wanted to use her therapy to examine these repetitive patterns in her relationship.

She was drawn to nursing, in part, because she struggled with an autoimmune illness throughout her childhood. She explained that she still felt a sense of physical vulnerability, which helped her feel compassion for other people who struggle. She planned to work in a children's hospital someday.

During one of our initial sessions, Heather explained, "It's hard for me to trust my body. I sort of feel detached from it much of the time. Maybe I'm angry with my body. I don't know, but I definitely got tired of feeling sick. I spent so many years being the sick one. Everyone in the family would be, like, 'What's next?!' I felt that way, too, actually. I was always sick with something. My health issues impacted everyone. I ruined family vacations more than once, and I know I kept my sister awake because there were periods when my mother needed to check on me through the night. I used to have night terrors. I would feel like something was chasing me. Kind of a big dark blob. I could never see what it was, but I still remember exactly what it felt like. It was terrifying."

"You shared a room with your sister, and she felt burdened by your night terrors?" I asked.

Heather hastened to come to her sister's defense. "To be fair, life was hard for my sister. I had so many issues. She was the healthy one. My mother was always paying so much attention to me. I know my sister felt neglected. It wasn't just the nightmares. I would have trouble breathing sometimes, and my mother would give me breathing treatments with a nebulizer. I also had several incidents of anaphylactic shock. One was from a wasp sting. That ended a family vacation in Montana when I was ten. Another time was when I ate shellfish while we were on a trip in Vancouver when I was seven."

"Those sound like very scary experiences."

"They totally derailed the vacations."

"Heather, there will be times when I interrupt you. I promise I won't do it often, and I won't do it unless I feel like it's really important to our work. This is one of those times. Did you notice that your reaction to your experiences of anaphylactic shock was different from my reaction?"

As if she was ready to continue in the same vein, Heather said, "I just feel really sad about how much of a burden I was."

"I understand that," I interjected, "and that's fine. I'm really glad you're telling me how you feel about it. Would you indulge me for a minute and just confirm that you heard how I reacted to your having experienced anaphylactic shock twice in your childhood while on vacations?"

"You said they must have been scary."

"Great. Thank you. I feel much better now. Kidding aside, we don't have to discuss the difference right now, but I do want you to hear it and to try to be curious about that difference—the difference not only between our descriptions of the events but also the difference between how I treated you and how you treated you." I told this to Heather because I could already see that she was in the habit of dismissing her needs. It's not unusual for someone who had special needs as a child to feel the need to compensate for that later in life. I wanted Heather to start to notice this self-neglect because it tends to contribute to a number of problems that we address in psychotherapy. As we rejoin my conversation with Heather, you will notice she continued in the thought pattern she had been exhibiting. This, also, isn't unusual. It takes time to change these patterns. The change process begins with noticing them.

Heather continued, "Well, mostly I just feel embarrassed about those experiences. I remember being in the emergency room in Vancouver. Even though my mom had the EpiPen, I needed to be taken to the ER. I remember when we went to sleep that night, my sister told me she thought I was faking because I had eaten scallops before. And she was right. I mean, I had eaten scallops. That really bothered me. Like, for years. When I told my mom what my sister had said, my sister got grounded, but I secretly felt totally confused by it. I kind of agreed with my sister, even though I knew I wasn't faking. I felt like I should have known, even though I couldn't have. Anyway, it wasn't until I was nineteen that I learned a kid can develop an allergy even if they never had it before. But for years I just felt so guilty. Like I was a burden to everyone."

"Do you ever feel that way with David?" I asked.

"Yes. I definitely annoy him. Sometimes I don't even realize what I did. The other night I was out with my friend Sheri at a happy hour. At about 6:30 p.m., I texted David. I knew he was in an evening class and he'd be out at seven. Sometimes he worries about me, so I texted him saying I'd be with Sheri until after he got home, and that I'd call him when I got home, later that night. So, Sheri and I had a nice time. At about 8:30, we're getting ready to leave. She goes to the bathroom. While I'm waiting for the check, I take out my phone and I see, like, twenty-five messages from David. He was asking me over and over where I was. In some texts, he was accusing me of lying. He was saying random stupid things like telling me happy hour ends at eight. So I called him, right there at the table, and he was so annoyed with me. I kept having to convince him I wasn't lying. When I got home, I called him again, and that seemed to help him. But we talked for about two hours. At one point, he told me he knew all along that I wasn't lying because he drove to the restaurant and saw my car there. He gets so worked up sometimes."

Heather explained that David was often deeply suspicious of her. He would also expect her to wait on him hand and foot when they were together. It was clearly an unequal, abusive relationship.

I commented to Heather once, "It seems like David is really demanding of you and not very nurturing. Is that the way you see his behavior?"

"I know he seems that way a lot. Sometimes when I tell you stories about him, I hear myself, and it causes me to think about it all more. Like, sometimes I feel like David behaves the way Mike did, the guy I dated before him. But Mike really had problems. He was an alcoholic, and when he'd get drunk he would be really out of control. He had a bad temper. David isn't violent."

"Heather, I'm curious to know what you think about something. Given what you told me about your childhood, do you have thoughts about how we can use your past to better understand your relationship dynamics with David?"

"I'm not sure. I mean, David's last girlfriend was dishonest. He caught her lying a bunch of times, and it led him to become a really untrusting person. He's still kind of getting over not being able to trust a girlfriend, you know?"

"Do you see how inclined you are to try to see what's bothering David? To see things from his perspective, I mean?"

"Well," Heather replied, "I want to be supportive."

I wanted to know whether Heather was seeing her pattern of choosing guys who treated her like she owed them something but they didn't owe her anything. She was treated by these guys as though she was a burden to have around, as though she needed to make up for the burden she was. That was why she was so inclined to accept their neglect and abuse. At this point in the treatment, Heather wasn't articulating an awareness of this.

She needed to recover from some painful childhood experiences. She also needed to see that, in some prominent ways, she was not taking good care of herself. This was especially true of her romantic relationships, David included. As a psychologist, I often look for ways to hold up a mirror for a client. In Heather's case, I needed to help her see her value. She needed to stop thinking of herself as a burden to the world. She needed to stop apologizing for her existence. She needed to see that she deserved to be loved and nurtured just because of who she is, not because of what she did for others. And she needed to see her strengths.

Heather's psychotherapy is relevant to the subject of cosmetic surgery because while I was working with her, she happened to mention she was planning to have lip and cheekbone injections. As if Heather needed to give me more reasons not to be one of David's biggest fans, she told me that David was not only an enthusiastic supporter of those intentions, but that he had given her the ideas.

I believed it would have been a mistake, aesthetically, for Heather to have undergone either of those procedures. And since I can't show you a picture of Heather, let me just add that I am confident almost anyone other than David would agree with me. But, of course, my job is not to presume to tell a client what clothing, makeup, or cosmetic procedure would or would not make them more attractive. I have no training or expertise in that regard. Besides, Heather wasn't asking for that kind of help. So, I needed to refrain from expressing any view.

Fortunately, her income prevented her from undergoing the procedures at least until after graduation. That was about a year away. I admit it—I secretly hoped our work would lead her to reexamine the intended procedures before that time came. I also hoped to help her question her tendency to accept inequality in her romantic relationships.

The Epiphany

Heather was as bright as she was humble. She worked hard in her therapy, and her keen insights helped her make quick progress. She implemented a daily loving kindness meditation, and she used her journal weekly. As a science-minded person, the direct and logical approach to psychotherapy resonated with her. She began asking David to notice her needs more often. More and more she noticed the inequalities in their relationship, and she began setting limits with him. I was pleasantly surprised to hear that her new behaviors seemed to have a gradual impact on David's behavior. That is, I was not surprised Heather made progress, but I was surprised David seemed to be changing.

Heather still had difficulty asserting herself without apologizing for it. She didn't allow herself to occupy much space in the world. She tended to keep her needs to herself. A great example of this emerged during one of our sessions. Heather was describing her week as relatively uneventful when she mentioned that she did have an "unusual" experience. "Do you want to tell me about it?" I asked.

She casually replied, "Oh, sure. I don't feel like there's a reason to tell you, except that it was unusual. I was walking with my friend Gail. We were going by this park. It was about three o'clock, last Thursday. So, we hear this screeching sound like tires on pavement, and then the sound of metal scraping. When we looked, we saw a motorcycle and the rider flying through the air, separately. He fell and hit something and flew up in the air and then fell down and skidded and bounced and rolled and somehow ended up actually in the park. I went over and asked him if he was okay. He didn't reply or move, and his posture was really unnatural. I called over to Gail and told her to call 911. I guess his helmet wasn't strapped on, because it was off and he hit his head on something. Gail can't stand blood, so she was, like, fifty feet away. He was bleeding a lot. You could see it running on the sidewalk. I tried to wake him up, but I didn't want to move him, because I didn't know how he fell or what could be hurt. The 911 operator started asking questions. The medical person on the phone said it sounded like I needed to do more until they arrived. So, I described what I saw, and Gail relayed what I said, and they walked me through what to do. They were worried his airway needed to be opened, so I had to move his head. And he had a really deep gash on his forehead. It was pouring blood. They said I needed to apply pressure to it, but that I needed to try not to put pressure on his neck. It was hard, because he wasn't moving, and his head was really slippery from all the blood."

"So, did you just have your hand on the wound?" I asked, totally engrossed in the dramatic scene she was describing.

"At first, but it was too slippery," Heather said. "I had a polyester scarf, so I switched to that. Luckily, the ambulance got there in about five or ten minutes, but it felt like forever. I was covered in blood. It got under my nails, it was in my hair, it dripped onto my shoes—it was everywhere. The ambulance driver told me I needed to throw out all of my clothes and wash myself very carefully right when I got home, because the blood might be dangerous. Luckily the police took me home, because I'd have gotten Gail's car all bloody." Heather concluded her story by saying, again, very casually and without a hint of sarcasm, "Like I said, I don't really have a reason for telling you about it except that it happened."

My first thought was to check on how Heather was doing. An incident like this can be traumatizing, even if the client is unaware that it had that impact. I needed to be sure Heather wasn't experiencing symptoms of post-traumatic stress disorder (PTSD). "I'm glad you decided to tell me about it, Heather. Can I ask you some questions?"

"Sure," Heather said.

"Have you been thinking about it much? For instance, have you been replaying it in your mind?"

Heather indicated she had not been thinking about the incident. When asked, she also told me that she hadn't had any dreams about it, either. And she denied any experience of feeling anxious or jumpy since the incident. She also denied any avoidance of things associated with the event. I saw no evidence of PTSD caused by the incident.

After answering my questions, Heather said, "I do wonder if the guy is okay. I don't even know where he was taken. I didn't think to ask. It all happened so fast."

"And you mentioned that Gail doesn't deal well with blood, right?"

"Yeah, she couldn't look at all. I was worried she would get sick when I described his wounds. His head was in really bad shape. The gash was really deep, and I had to describe it."

As Heather told the story, she was completely calm. In her mind, there was nothing special about what she did. This was true even though she had the clear counterexample of her friend, Gail, who couldn't have done any of the things Heather did for that biker.

Psychologically, we tend to think of ourselves in particular ways. How we define ourselves remains fairly stable. The definition we choose comes from various factors, including our own view of ourselves and also how other people in our lives have treated us and described us. This all contributes to what psychologists call our self-concept—the person we view ourselves to be. We carry that self-concept into different settings in our life.

Heather's tone reflected her view of herself in a way that was breathtaking, to me. She simply could not see herself as powerful and brave and heroic, even though her actions on that day revealed all those qualities. She couldn't see them because they were inconsistent with the person she had always believed herself to be.

When she finished telling the story, I felt consumed by it all. I was processing what I'd heard as I was observing Heather. Finally I spoke up. "Heather, I think you just told me that since our most recent session, you saved someone's life."

Heather replied without hesitation, "Well, I was just the one who was there. And really, I just followed their instructions. If the 911 or EMS people on the phone hadn't been there, I would never have known what to do."

"Can I ask you to pay close attention to what you're doing right now? Do you notice?"

"I'm just saying the truth is I don't even know if he is alive. I might not have accomplished anything for him."

"I understand." I paused and held my gaze on her for a beat. When I continued, I wanted to be direct but still gentle and supportive. "Is it possible you're minimizing what you did, Heather?"

"I guess," she said. "I just never thought of it that way—that I saved his life."

"I think that's an important insight: you never thought of it that way. Let me ask you something: if Gail had been walking through the park alone that day, would she have done what you did?"

Heather looked at me as if I was confused. "Gail could barely *breathe*. She was about to faint the whole time. She was sure she was going to vomit. I had to drag her close enough to me to relay the descriptions to the medical person on the phone so they could help me help him."

"So, as you describe Gail, I think you know you're describing the way a lot of people would have responded. The blood, the unconscious guy, the uncertainty of how to follow the instructions from the EMS people, the possibility of doing something wrong—all of it would have been too much for many people. But it wasn't too much for you. You were able to remain completely present and on task. It's pretty extraordinary."

Heather stopped and thought for a moment. "I guess. I'm kind of uncomfortable hearing that. I'm not sure why."

"It's so great that you notice that. Try to allow yourself to be curious about the discomfort. About where it comes from within you."

We sat quietly for a minute or two. The session was drawing to a close, and I wanted to address something before stopping. "Heather, can I say something else that occurs to me?" She nodded and I continued, "Another thing I can't stop thinking about is this: you learned something about yourself that day. You learned what's inside you. Most of us never learn for sure whether we have that courage inside us. We all hope we do. We hope that, if a sudden crisis were to happen, we would have the capacity to act. But the truth is, trauma is unpredictable. Until the crisis is upon us, we really can't know whether we have that strength and ability within us. Because of this incident, now you know. It's quite a gift, Heather."

Heather sat with this. "I think I need to think about this some more," she finally said.

"I agree. Let's discuss this more, next time."

In the months that followed, Heather and I examined how this incident altered the way she viewed herself. In the process, she realized she had always seen herself as a vulnerable person. She had always dated young men with dominant personalities. Her persona with everyone was that of the sweet, polite woman who needed to be cared for and protected, especially by men. This incident enabled her to begin to question that. She began seeing the ways she had always minimized her accomplishments.

Heather made a lot of progress. She began asserting herself in different settings in her life. Her family and friends noticed the changes in her. More and more, she was allowing her voice to be heard.

She continued dating David. He was a work in progress, but their relationship seemed to be evolving in positive ways. And I'm most happy to report that she decided not to go through with the cosmetic work.

Self-Confidence and Tolerating Risk

It's true Heather was considering undergoing multiple cosmetic services, but there is another reason I decided to discuss Heather's treatment within this section addressing risk tolerance. Her actions in helping that biker occurred within the context of considerable uncertainty. She couldn't possibly have known whether she would succeed. She had no idea how to help, and she had no crisis response experience or training. And yet she acted.

I hope you can use Heather's experience to help you nurture your ability to tolerate the risk that your procedure will not go as planned. Heather showed what a person can do if they don't allow doubts and uncertainty to dictate their actions. She felt very much attached to the vulnerable part of herself, yet she was able to set it aside when she needed to. She reminds us that we can push ourselves to confront risks, even if we feel vulnerable.

Maybe you, like Heather, have more of a capacity to confront risk than you typically think you do. At the end of this chapter, there is a journaling exercise called "You Tolerate Risk Every Day." The objective of the exercise is to give you practice realizing how often you tolerate risk, and how you do it. It's a simple exercise that nevertheless has helped a number of clients recognize their strengths. You may choose to do it once, or several times a week, leading up to the day of your procedure. I hope you will try it. It's so important for every patient preparing for a cosmetic procedure to believe in their ability to tolerate risk.

Specific Risks

The remainder of this chapter will be dedicated to identifying specific sources of risk and discussing ways of coping with them. Please note: some of the content in the remainder of this chapter is medically explicit and might trigger some readers to worry excessively. If you struggle with an anxiety disorder, it may be best for you to read the remainder of this chapter with a mental health professional who can help you process your reactions in healthy ways.

The "Risk" of Imperfection

Cosmetic patients often have perfectionistic expectations. They pursue the cosmetic work with a particular objective. Given that cosmetic outcomes are never completely predictable, the patient is required to cope with quite a stressful situation.

The desire for predictability in surgical outcomes can be particularly intense for patients who are public figures. Often, these people's livelihood depends on the procedure achieving certain specified goals. To make matters worse, the patients often are aware that there are other people to please; agents, managers, directors, or other artists may also be relying on the procedure's success.

Patients need to manage their anxiety over the unpredictability of these procedures. One way for the patient to do this is to first articulate the elements of a successful outcome. I encourage clients to do this in writing. Once it's clear what the patient seeks, it's helpful for them to bring the description of their goal to the surgeon to obtain confirmation regarding the likelihood of their desired outcome. Typically, after discussing these issues with the surgeon, patients return to my office with a much more balanced set of expectations. The important thing is for patients to feel confident that the outcome sought is reasonably likely to be achieved, despite the reality that outcomes cannot be guaranteed.

Independent Research Risks

Remember the way James compulsively researched before-and-after images? We discussed his tendency to plan for worst-case scenarios, as well as his discomfort with uncertainty and failure. Those behaviors are all commonly exhibited in someone struggling with anxiety. Just as James became lost in the process of looking at before-and-after photos, any cosmetic patient can devote an excessive amount of attention to other aspects of the process of choosing the right surgeon and procedure.

Acquiring accurate information is an important aspect of coping with anxiety. I often advise clients to conduct careful research. It's helpful for them to learn as much as they can about any issues that contribute to their anxiety.

One way patients can acquire valuable information is by consulting physicians they already know. When a patient can consult their own surgeon, the way Elliot did, that usually brings the added benefit of further reassuring the client about their own surgeon's knowledge and expertise.

A second way to conduct research is through targeted online searches of *knowledgeable, professionally written, or peer-reviewed articles.* Try to find articles approved by medical centers. The National Institutes of Health, the Mayo Clinic, and the Cleveland Clinic are usually valuable resources. So are medical and cosmetic surgery journals. For information specific to cosmetic procedures, the websites for the American Board of Plastic Surgery and the American Board of Cosmetic Surgery are both excellent sources. Meanwhile, be wary of "branded" or "native" content—information provided and sponsored by a person or company that stands to benefit from informing you. A few ways to identify biased sources are to note the website address, who is quoted, and the sources of the information.

I always warn patients about acquiring information from other patients. Patients should not be relied upon for substantive information. Leave that to the verifiably unbiased and informed sources. Another patient can, however, provide useful firsthand information about the subjective aspects of a procedure: how the doctor treated them, how the surgery went, what they liked or didn't like.

If you read patient accounts, be mindful of how you do it. Evaluate their accounts as you would evaluate anything that is inherently subjective, like a book or music review. In patient accounts, focus on the emotional experience more than facts and figures because their subjective experience as a patient is really the most reliable thing they have to offer you. This is why it's best that you rely on the experts, surgeons, and types of sources I mentioned earlier for your core information.

Risk of Surgical Complications

Cosmetic surgery patients often focus excessively on surgical complications. Effective psychotherapy can typically provide rapid help with this tendency. Initially, it's always important to acknowledge that being aware of risks is healthy. After all, complications are part of our reality. But it's also important for the client to recognize the positive pieces of information that help them cope with the risks. For instance:

- Major surgical complications are relatively rare.
- Surgeons can help us recover from complications in many ways.
- A surgeon's instructions make complications less likely.

- Surgical complications are often only temporary.

- A surgeon's instructions make complications less serious.

- We can cope with surgical complications.

These are all examples of how the cognitive aspect of the work in psychotherapy is pretty straightforward. Ultimately, it's all about helping the client view their entire reality, rather than just the negative pieces. In this way, we seek to use psychotherapy to enhance the accuracy of the patient's mindset, helping them think in more balanced, healthy, and empowered ways.

Physiological Risks

A glance at any drug label reminds us that medical interventions can affect our body in a variety of ways, both positive and negative. As a psychologist, I can assist cosmetic patients in weighing various potential physiological risks associated with a procedure. In doing that work, I do not offer medical advice or information because those types of help lie outside my area of expertise. Likewise, it exceeds the scope of this book to discuss all the medical risks attached to various procedures. So I want to offer this important piece of advice: *explore all possible risks with your physician, and seek additional medical advice from qualified sources until all your medical questions and concerns have been addressed.*

There are a number of common general surgical complications you may want to discuss ahead of time with a physician. By consulting a book on the subject, you can explore these issues at your own pace and without the difficulty of finding a surgeon willing to consult with you. A number of physicians have written really informative books on this subject. One that I often recommend to clients is *The Essential Cosmetic Surgery Companion*, by Robert Kotler, MD. Another really comprehensive medical resource is *Straight Talk About Cosmetic Surgery*, by Arthur Perry, MD.

To help you explore the risk profile of a given procedure, I've compiled a list of potential complications patients have discussed during psychotherapy sessions. You can use this checklist to assist you to identify issues that concern you. Any risk that feels relevant can and should be discussed with your surgeon. For each item of concern, you will want to not only explore the likelihood that the complication could occur but also the treatment and recovery options.

Risk List

1. Problems related to anesthesia

2. Infections

3. Bruising

4. Ongoing pain conditions

5. Nerve damage beyond what is expected

6. Damage to blood vessels, muscles, lungs, or other internal organs

7. Postoperative bleeding

8. Scarring/poor wound healing

9. Cardiac complications

10. Pulmonary complications, including those due to blood clots

11. Hematomas (internal bleeding)

12. Numbness

13. Nausea

14. Incorrect positioning of implants

15. Implant leakage/rupture

16. Fluid accumulation

17. Skin wrinkling

18. Heat injuries

19. Asymmetry

20. Irregular pigmentation

21. Various less-common risks associated with particular surgical procedures

22. Psychiatric complications

Interviewing Your Surgeon about Risks

We have explored the reasons why it's normal to feel anxiety prior to surgery. And we've noted that one helpful tool for coping with anxiety is obtaining accurate information regarding how likely surgical complications are, and also identifying ways to cope with them if they do arise. At the end of this chapter, there is an exercise called "Interviewing Your Surgeon About Risks." The exercise is designed to assist you to discuss these issues with your surgeon and thereby gain confidence in your ability to cope with the uncertainty.

Risk of Death

In extreme and very rare cases, surgical complications can lead to death. That's the ultimate risk for any surgery, really. Fortunately, the likelihood that a cosmetic service will result in death is very low.

This subject is yet another that reminds us of the value of confronting our fears. Remember: one of the most empowering tools for managing fear is accurate information. In this instance, that means learning about the true risk of death associated with your procedure. For this information, your surgeon would be the most helpful initial source to consult. Your surgeon should be open to addressing your questions directly. Related concerns that involve the anesthesia process can be directed to your anesthesiologist. If, after consulting your physicians and other sources of information, you find you are still struggling to feel safe, you might want to talk with a mental health professional to help you explore whether there are psychological factors impacting your process of coping with the risk of death.

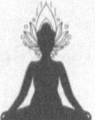

Exercise: You Tolerate Risk Every Day

This is a quick journaling exercise that can help you gain clarity about your ability to cope with risk. When I suggest this exercise to clients, I encourage them to be brief in their responses. This exercise is especially helpful when repeated several times, so I tell clients to try not to over-think their responses. If you choose to do it, I think you will find it empowering as well as clarifying.

1. An hour before bedtime, ideally at the same time each night, sit with your journal.

2. Create a table like the one below, with three columns.

   Label the left column "Situation Calling for Action," the center column "Possible Outcomes" and the right column "Reasons I Was Able to Act."

Situation Calling for Action	Possible Outcomes	Reasons I Was Able to Act

3. Name any two things that occurred today that required you to act without complete knowledge of the consequences.

As you answer this question, it's good to have the right mindset. First, as you do the exercise, try to remain mindful that its purpose is to show you that you do act in the face of uncertainty throughout every day. Second, as you fill in your table, think broadly. Every single day, without advanced preparation, you respond in the moment to circumstances you could not possibly have predicted. At those times, you accept that the consequences of your actions are somewhat unpredictable. In this exercise, you will choose two of those situations. These might involve big decisions you made in your workplace or at home. More likely, you'll see that most of the things on this list will not be so momentous. Consider, for instance, the ways you responded in a split second when a decision was needed—while commuting (choosing this route over that one, this lane over that one, and so on), in a market or a restaurant (choosing what to eat, sometimes immediately after learning that your first choice was no longer available), or perhaps in brief social interactions (choosing what to say or where to look).

Sample Table:

Situation Calling for Action	Possible Outcomes	Reasons I Was Able to Act
I needed to choose a sandwich from the list at the new restaurant.	I could have disliked sandwich #4 or I could have loved it.	It's only one lunch. Next time I will choose the other sandwich if I didn't like the one I chose.
I needed to speak with X about his performance on project Y.	X might have reacted very angrily to my questions about project Y, or X could have felt frightened and intimidated by me and closed up.	I cannot control his reactions. I knew I was doing what I believed was best, and that's all that matters.
I told my project partner Emma that joke.	Emma might have laughed and our work relationship might have improved, or Emma might have thought it was not funny or appropriate to tell her the joke at work.	It's good to get along with co-workers. I had a good intention.

Note that column 3 is intended to be a rational, reassuring, friendly explanation for your behavior. The objective is to take a moment and tell yourself something that helps you to move on instead of ruminating about whatever happened after you acted in a particular way when an outcome was not completely predictable.

Interviewing Your Surgeon about Risks

Listed below are questions you can ask your surgeon to address some common concerns. The answers will assist you in your process of evaluating the risks and benefits associated with a procedure, given your unique medical history and current condition.

1. What are the risks commonly associated with this procedure? How often do they occur?

2. What are the risks less commonly associated with this procedure? How often do they occur?

3. Under what circumstances might the common risks appear? In other words, what makes these more likely? What can I do to reduce the likelihood that any of these will occur?

4. How are these complications treated when they occur?

5. Do any of my current medical conditions or past medical conditions increase the likelihood that I will experience any of these complications?

6. Are any of these complications untreatable? If so, how might a person's future health and lifestyle be impacted?

7. Would any of my past or current medical conditions limit my options for treatment for any of these complications?

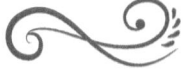

CHAPTER 10

When Flowers Need More than Water

Peace comes from within.
Do not seek it without.

— Buddha

Transformation

From a psychological perspective, some people are not good candidates for cosmetic surgery—at least not without first engaging in effective psychotherapy. For these patients, this type of procedure runs a higher risk of failing. Whenever any medical procedure fails, it's difficult and disappointing. When the failed procedure is cosmetic, and when the patient is psychologically frail, the psychological consequences of the failure are compounded.

We've explored the transformational power of certain cosmetic surgical work. The problem is some patients have an unhealthy need for transformation. They have devoted their entire lives to directing unfair criticisms at themselves. These patients seek a surgery-induced cosmetic change to transform much more than aspects of their appearance. They often seek to achieve dramatic transformations in their social and psychological identities as well.

Psychological research has repeatedly examined this issue and has warned that some cosmetic surgery patients are unlikely to feel satisfied. This raises several important questions:

1. Which cosmetic surgery patients are unlikely to feel satisfied?

2. How can you determine whether you are one of those patients?

3. If you are one of those patients, what can you do to become a patient who is more likely to feel satisfied after a cosmetic procedure?

Appearance Matters

Greg was a thirty-two-year-old man who was using psychotherapy to overcome the condition known as body dysmorphic disorder (BDD). BDD is characterized by an overly critical focus on one's own perceived physical flaws. A common misconception is that BDD is a problem only for women. Men struggle with BDD, too. Though it's considered slightly more common in women, I suspect the difference is due more to research design deficits than it is to true gender differences in BDD.

In one session, Greg spoke about a typical childhood experience. "When I was about fourteen, my aunt Ethel came over. I was in the living room watching TV. When she entered the room, she said, "Gregory, you are getting so handsome." I remember feeling paralyzed in that moment. I was a shy kid, but it was more than that. I'd spend hours studying myself in the mirror. I hated how I looked. My hair was never quite right, my teeth were never white enough, and my skin was never clear enough. There were always blemishes to pick at, hairs to cut or pull, and things to do to my teeth to try to make them whiter and cleaner.

"So, when my Aunt Ethel said that to me, I heard her compliment as confirmation of my ugliness. I assumed she was just being nice to help me not feel so bad about how I looked. I was convinced she was just a big liar. I absolutely hated it when she came to the house. I avoided her like the plague."

Greg managed his appearance compulsively. He also evaluated other people, especially those who noticed anything about the way he looked. He carefully scrutinized anything related to his appearance. He engaged in a lot of what psychologists refer to as comparing and despairing. He compared his current self to his past selves, he compared himself to people he knew or to famous people, and he even compared himself to inanimate objects like mannequins and anime characters. Like many people with his tendency to be so self-critical, he knew he was being unfair to himself, but he couldn't stop.

We've all had moments when we felt the sting of someone's judgment. For people like Greg, the struggle is different, occurring not daily, but hourly. The search for flaws is an obsession and the need to correct ones that are located is a compulsion. It becomes like an addiction. The need to look for flaws and to correct them is irresistible and unquenchable. It is a kind of perfectionism.

We all can imagine improved and enhanced images of ourselves. In this age of Photoshop and other methods of digital editing, we are encouraged to strive for perfection. It's common to see images of beautiful people who appear flawless.

In addition to the images we see in the media, we are also impacted by the people closest to us. Well-meaning friends, family members, and even strangers continually encourage us to evaluate the way we look. Even the well-intentioned Aunt Ethels of the world are letting us know that they are looking at us, and that their opinion should matter to us. These influences often cause people to focus excessively on their appearance and to search desperately for defects.

Is it any wonder that the pursuit of attractiveness can diminish self-confidence and self-esteem? For many people, thoughts about their perceived physical flaws are compulsive and create debilitating self-consciousness. Like any form of perfectionism, the result is not that the person feels closer to perfect. *The result of any perfectionism is a reinforcement of a feeling of inadequacy.* Without an effective intervention, people like Greg continue to be harshly critical of their appearance, often with growing intensity.

Divide and Conquer?

People who look at themselves excessively tend to focus on particular aspects that they wish were different. For these people, looking into the mirror becomes an obsessive and abusive activity. Some people invest years of their lives into chasing physical ideals. This often involves segmenting the body into parts, resulting in statements I've heard from clients such as, "I love the changes I made to my nose, but my cheekbones seem too rounded." Or, "I like how flat my stomach is, but my upper arms are too flabby." Or "My new square jaw is just what I wanted, but now I need to add a dimple to my chin." The desire to change one's appearance can be self-reinforcing. It can be hard to know when to stop.

Why is it often so difficult to know when to stop pursuing cosmetic surgery? The answer usually lies in the patient's reasons for seeking the procedures. Within the physical changes the patient seeks is a set of expectations about how the changes will alter the ways other people treat them.

It's not unhealthy to want other people to treat you well. And it isn't unhealthy to recognize that people might treat you differently if you change the way you look. These things acquire their unhealthy and abusive quality when they inhabit the mind of a person who is habitually self-abusive. Many people have difficulty being kind to themselves. It's a subject we don't discuss enough. But some people have that problem to an even greater degree.

People who struggle with a sense of inadequacy tend to seek affirmation from others because they get so little from themselves. Some people seeking cosmetic improvements have this problem: they feel a desire to be seen differently in the hope that it will help them see *themselves* differently.

For several reasons, cosmetic patients who suffer in these ways are less likely to find satisfaction in cosmetic procedures. The first problem is that they mistakenly think they have an attractiveness deficit. Even without seeing them I can tell you this isn't their main problem. Their main problem lies in their self-image and the choice they make to habitually mistreat themselves. No cosmetic service will reverse that.

Another reason these patients are likely to feel unsatisfied with the procedure is that they can, if they choose to. Cosmetic outcomes are always subjective. You may wonder why a patient would choose to feel unsatisfied. In this instance, the choice would be more due to habit than to a conscious decision. To understand the reason for the habit, consider this statement attributed to Groucho Marx: "I don't want to belong to any club that would admit me as one of its members." People who have always struggled with a sense of inadequacy have devoted years to seeing themselves as flawed. As a result, they often feel like attractive clothing does not look attractive when they wear the items. Like the club that admits them, whatever attaches itself to the person loses desirability in that person's eyes.

When someone who has this problem undergoes a cosmetic procedure, the problem is any cosmetic change is attached to the patient. This is why there is a very real possibility that a habitually self-critical patient will be unsatisfied with any cosmetic outcome.

These are some of the reasons a patient who relies on a cosmetic procedure to improve self-esteem is destined to feel disappointed. It's not unhealthy to enjoy being admired by others, but it is unhealthy if you feel you need that external admiration in order to admire yourself. Inner growth and the development of self-love should be pursued apart from, and prior to, the cosmetic surgical work.

When the Issue Is More than Just Low Self-Esteem

Some people who seek a cosmetic procedure have, for years, oppressed themselves with thoughts of their own inadequacy. These negative ways of thinking often focus not only on rejection of parts of their body, but also on the type of person they view themselves to be. The thoughts tend to center on personal inadequacy, and they typically repeat, in a never-ending, self-reinforcing, negative feedback loop.

You may wonder why the feedback loop would be self-reinforcing. The answer is it's always possible to find flaws. Whether a person is judging their performance or their appearance, the judgment is always subjective. When the judgment is made, a flaw will inevitably be discovered, because everything has flaws in the eyes of the observer who is looking for them.

You may be thinking that finding flaws is a success strategy. That's true when it is moderated by reasonableness. The people who struggle in the way I'm describing don't moderate their demands. They make a habit of embracing overly narrow and rigid demands on themselves. As a result, they suffer deeply.

Kathy was such a person. An attractive twenty-eight-year-old Certified Financial Planner, she succeeded professionally despite being preoccupied by excessive concerns about her complexion. Although she did have some acne scars on her face, they were relatively minor. The problem is, she would continually create new ones by compulsively picking at any imperfection. In an average evening, she would devote hours to staring into the mirror and picking at blemishes. Her preoccupation led her to miss out on social gatherings, which in turn impacted her ability to acquire new clients. Her social and romantic relationships were affected because she never felt worthy of positive romantic attention.

Dr. D, a psychologically-minded dermatologist, referred Kathy to me. She had consulted him about cosmetic improvements. Dr. D knew there were procedures that would correct some of Kathy's complexion issues. Fortunately, however, Dr. D recognized that Kathy's compulsive picking at her skin revealed deeper struggles that would likely undermine any skillful cosmetic work Dr. D could provide.

Like Greg, Kathy's psychotherapy focused on helping her conquer body dysmorphic disorder (BDD). After reading about Greg, you may recognize that BDD treatment focuses on the person's unhealthy and inaccurate perception of the way parts of their body look and their preoccupation with the need to substantially change those parts. You may also have observed that people who suffer in this way often struggle with co-occurring mental health conditions such as anxiety, depression, bipolar disorder, substance abuse, or eating disorders. These can intensify the struggle with BDD and can lead to a self-destructive reliance on cosmetic surgery in an effort to overcome a deeply felt sense of inadequacy. The effort is destined to fail.

During the psychotherapy process, I strongly encourage clients like Kathy to continue the work between sessions. This is often accomplished through manageable exercises we design together. Some clients are drawn to great self-help books. Two exceptional ones that I recommend to clients are *The Body Image Workbook*, by Thomas Cash, PhD and *Feeling Good About The Way You Look*, by Sabine Wilhelm, PhD. I'm sure the brief screeners I created were inspired not only by my own professional reading and clinical work but also by ideas and methods provided in great self-help resources I've found for clients (a more comprehensive list of resources can be found in Appendix A).

Kathy compulsively and intensely inspected her image in the mirror, constantly searching for imperfections. Her focus invariably landed on skin blemishes. If she were to find one, she would take extreme measures to eliminate it. She had acquired a large collection of expensive drying creams for acne, lightening creams for freckles, and various masks. She also owned several tools that enabled her to cut off moles or skin tags, or physically manipulate blemishes in her efforts to hasten their elimination. Dr. D had warned Kathy many times that the tools she acquired should only be used by trained professionals. He explicitly told her she must never cut her skin, because it could cause a dangerous infection.

None of Dr. D's warnings deterred Kathy, until one of Kathy's cutting incidents led to a life-threatening infection. Ironically, Kathy's concern about eliminating skin imperfections that she believed made her look sickly created a serious infection that literally threatened her life. This was when Kathy was referred to me.

Kathy suffered from a long history of self-abuse. Talking with her, I felt as though she was caught in a whirlpool caused by the cyclical, self-perpetuating nature of her behaviors, thoughts, and feelings. For many years she had exhibited a tendency to feel self-doubt, be overly self-critical, and make excessive demands on herself. All of these compelled her to focus on her skin blemishes. The habits grew more and more intense until they culminated with the life-threatening infection.

The tendency to criticize your own appearance can be deceptively powerful. I've seen a number of clients who don't even realize they are abusing themselves. This is why I strongly recommend that, if any of the descriptions of Kathy's struggles resonate with your experiences, even if your struggle is much milder than Kathy's, you should explore that with a mental health professional prior to pursuing any cosmetic surgical procedure.

Should You Talk with a Mental Health Professional?

Before leaving the subject of BDD, I want to provide you another simple screening tool. Like the Appearance Self-Consciousness Measure (ASM), this tool will help you explore whether you should talk with a mental health professional about your body image concerns before undergoing a cosmetic surgical service. I call this screening tool the Body Image Concerns (BIC) Screener. The BIC Screener is not an assessment tool for diagnosing body dysmorphic disorder, nor is it a formal, empirically-validated, peer-reviewed psychological assessment tool. This is simply a brief screening tool I created to help prospective cosmetic surgery patients evaluate the way they view their body. I often use a patient's BIC results to guide my conversation with them in the initial phases of our work together.

I always remind clients that the purpose of the BIC is not to prevent anyone from pursuing a cosmetic procedure. The BIC is simply a way for you to gather information about the ways you currently view your body. You can use your BIC results to help guide you as you consider whether it would be helpful to talk with a mental health professional about your cosmetic surgery plans and your history of past procedures before moving forward with the plans.

The Body Image Concerns (BIC) Test

Directions: Please choose the response that best reflects your experience or mindset.

1. I look into the mirror to detect beauty defects...
   a. ...at least daily. (5)
   b. ...2 or 3 out of every 7 days. (3)
   c. ...no more than once a week. (1)
   d. I never do this. (-1)

2. I ask loved ones about flaws in my appearance...
   a. ...at least daily. (5)
   b. ...2 to 3 out of every 7 days. (3)
   c. ...no more than once a week. (1)
   d. I never do this. (-1)

3. I have had a cosmetic procedure to correct a past procedure...
   a. ...never. (0)
   b. ...once. (2)
   c. ...twice. (4)
   d. ...three times or more. (6)

4. I have had a cosmetic procedure that a different cosmetic surgeon had refused to perform on me...
   a. ...never. (0)
   b. ...once. (3)
   c. ...twice. (5)
   d. ...three times or more. (6)

5. The number of loved ones who have suggested that I've had too many cosmetic procedures is…
   a. …none. (0)
   b. …one. (2)
   c. …two. (4)
   d. …three or more. (6)

6. If I had unlimited resources, the total number of elements of my appearance I believe I would change surgically is…
   a. …0 to 1. (0)
   b. …2 to 3. (3)
   c. …4 to 5. (5)
   d. …5 or more. (6)

Scoring. To score the test, simply look to the number in the parentheses after each answer and add up all your scores from the six items. The total of all answers is your total test score. For example, if your responses were 1. a (5), 2. d (-1), 3. a (0), 4. b (3), 5. a (0), 6. b (3), your total score would be 10.

Total test score of 10 or above: Your responses **strongly indicate** you would benefit from talking with a mental health professional before agreeing to undergo a cosmetic procedure. A mental health professional can help you weigh your options and examine all the things you seek from the procedure(s) you are planning. It's likely you have too critical a view of your appearance. There is a high risk that if you undergo a cosmetic procedure now, you will find the results unsatisfying. Unsatisfying results are difficult for any patient, but they may be more unpleasant to you than they would need to be. The right kind of work with a skilled mental health professional will help prepare you better so that the chances of a difficult outcome will be dramatically reduced.

Total test score of 6–9: Prior to undergoing a cosmetic procedure, *you are advised* to talk with a mental health professional to examine your values and the intensity of your desire to change your appearance.

If you endorsed any item that was scored with a 4 or higher: you would *probably benefit* from talking with a mental health professional to examine your values and the intensity of your desire to change your appearance.

Total test score of 5 and below with no individual answer score of 4 or higher: although effective psychotherapy is always beneficial, your responses suggest that **there is not a pressing need** for you to consult with a mental health professional prior to pursuing a cosmetic procedure. Your responses are generally indicative of a normal level of concern regarding your appearance. None of us is perfect and, from time to time, we all consider changing our appearance in various ways, whether with a surgical procedure or via other means such as grooming, makeup, hairstyles, or clothing.

One final note on this subject. To get an even clearer picture of these issues, you might consider your BIC results along with your results from the Appearance Self-Consciousness Measure (ASM), presented earlier in the book. Bringing both to a session with a mental health professional would give you a lot of helpful material to discuss.

Walking Roses

In addition to BDD, there are personality characteristics that cause some patients to experience more frequent emotional difficulties. A general label we can use for these patients is "prickly." It's common for prickly people to react with excessive criticism and to feel disappointed by other people.

Prickly is a good descriptor because, in a certain way, prickly people are like roses. We feel drawn to roses, but when we approach them inattentively, we get a prompt and painful reminder of our error. Like roses, prickly people punish those who approach without exercising extreme care.

There are very good reasons that explain prickliness that I'll discuss later in this chapter. For now, the important point is cosmetic patients sometimes bring special emotional needs to their procedures. When those special needs have not been managed, the journey toward a satisfying outcome tends to be bumpier.

Patients who are prickly suffer from a deep-seated struggle that can undermine the surgical outcome regardless of the quality of the surgeon's work. This is why it's so important that prickliness be recognized well ahead of the procedure date. When prickliness is present, it's sometimes best to delay the procedure until the prickliness can be addressed in effective psychotherapy.

Simply Delightful—and Prickly

Alexis was a prickly patient. I had been treating her for three months when she began informing me of her cosmetic procedure plans. She was a forty-six-year-old divorced entrepreneur. She had been married to an executive in the entertainment business. They had one child, a daughter, who was then fifteen years old.

We had been working on her recovery from divorce and the challenges of co-parenting with her ex. We had developed a nice rapport. She knew that I liked and respected her. Although Alexis didn't focus much on her feelings of vulnerability, it seemed clear to me that she needed time to feel safe enough with me to tell me about the cosmetic work she was considering.

One day she informed me of her plan to "eliminate my resting bitch face." She explained that she believed the divorce had taken a toll on her appearance. Her face, in her view, had acquired a "scowl" in the prior year.

She sought help from Dr. K, in particular, because she had seen "amazing" results in two friends who had been treated by him. Alexis said Dr. K had "literally saved" her friend Sara's face.

"'Literally saved'?" I asked, playfully drawing attention to her language.

"You think I'm being dramatic," she replied. "I'm telling you, Sara had a nose like an English bulldog. You should see her now. Gorgeous. It's remarkable."

Even more impressive to Alexis was the work Dr. K did for Carole, another woman in her friend group. Alexis explained, "I don't know how he did it, but Dr. K corrected Carole's lip implants. They were monstrous. Obscene, even. I told her that. She needed a friend to tell her that she looked like she was dating a Dirt Devil."

I understood why people felt drawn to Alexis. She was a very funny woman. Her descriptions were always vivid. She seemed to have firm opinions on every subject, which she shared often and dramatically. She reminded me of a young Joan Rivers.

During his treatment of Alexis, Dr. K asked to speak with me about certain concerns he had. With her permission, I did that. He told me that, initially, he found Alexis to be delightful and endearing, if a bit dramatic. "She asked me to help her soften some of her facial features with a pretty minor filler procedure. I told her I thought it would be a good idea, a smart approach given the issue that concerned her. I performed the procedure, and everything seemed to have gone very well."

Dr. K performs filler procedures multiple times each week. As is his practice, during the week after the procedure, he recommended some minor and temporary lifestyle changes to Alexis in order to speed her recovery. He wanted her to return in a week to see how the filler had settled.

Dr. K later explained that, up to this point, Alexis seemed exceedingly satisfied. She had been very friendly toward the doctor's staff and even sent a dozen roses to the doctor's office later in the day, after her procedure.

Although Alexis initially felt satisfied, she called Dr. K's office at least once on each of the three days following her procedure. She returned to his office the next week and insisted on meeting with him. She believed her face had swollen and then healed in an unnatural way, creating new issues that needed to be corrected immediately.

While they discussed Alexis's concerns, her dissatisfaction seemed to intensify. "She told me I'd made her face oblong. She said she looked exactly like Quasimodo. Those were her words," Dr. K explained. "I told her she was seeing normal swelling and that the amount of swelling isn't entirely predictable. The truth is she did have more swelling than I would have expected at that point in the healing process. I wondered about that until she solved the mystery. She revealed that since the procedure she had several face massages. Face massages!" Now Dr. K's voice was raised. "I specifically told her no massages for a week. I assume, if anything, a patient might seek a body massage and her face would rest in the cushioned face holder, which could be bad. That can damage the filler work, so I explicitly tell all my patients not to get a massage until I see them in a week. But who would expect a patient to actually get a *facial* massage right after a filler treatment?! She ruined my work and she also delayed the healing."

Alexis insisted on injections to correct the new issues. Dr. K told Alexis she was suggesting too many procedures. He explained that there would be a risk of facial distortion if he were to do all of them. He suggested a more moderated approach involving removing the filler he had injected and starting again once her face recovered. Alexis didn't want to delay the correction.

Alexis was unsuccessful in her efforts to convince Dr. K to immediately provide her with additional facial fillers. When the doctor held firm, Alexis increased the pressure, accusing him of abandoning her. Distraught, she told him he had turned her into a "monster," at one point even accusing him of being "abusive." She also labeled him "arrogant." This was when she confided in one of Dr. K's assistants that she was being treated by me, which led Dr. K to call me.

Dr. K was rattled by Alexis's reactions. Since she was so unhappy, even when he offered to remove the filler he had injected, Dr. K made two suggestions. First, he suggested Alexis could seek a second opinion from a different cosmetic surgeon. Second, he informed Alexis that, before finalizing a plan to perform multiple cosmetic procedures on any patient, he generally insists that the patient discuss the plan with a psychotherapist. Since she was already seeing me, he suggested she discuss her idea with me.

I approved of this suggestion, particularly because Alexis and I had an established relationship. Between Dr. K's wise and patient response to her and my processing her reactions and concerns, we were able to help her defer to Dr. K. She followed his advice.

Unfortunately, with prickly patients, the situation often quickly devolves beyond the point of salvaging the relationship with the surgeon. Ideally, prickliness should be addressed prior to the initial procedure. After the initial procedure, an unhappy prickly patient is likely to resist the suggestion to consult with a psychologist.

Identifying and Helping the Prickly Patient

People who are not mental health providers might be surprised to learn that there are many people like Alexis. Despite being a talented and successful adult who was managing her life quite well, Alexis was coping with some chronic and fairly prominent untreated psychological issues. Her intellect and social adeptness concealed the emotional struggle.

It should not be surprising that psychological vulnerabilities are often concealed from cosmetic surgeons. Initial meetings with cosmetic surgeons are full of hope and encouragement. I'm not suggesting surgeons and their staff pitch procedures to patients (though some do) but rather that both the surgeons and the patients are eager to explore how the surgeon's skill and training can assist the patient to achieve cosmetic objectives.

Under those hopeful circumstances, psychological vulnerabilities are more likely to be understated or not mentioned. This isn't necessarily because patients want to lie (although some certainly do). On the contrary, normally, psychological vulnerabilities wax and wane and so they are often perceived by the sufferer to be issues that no longer plague them. This is often accurate in the sense that, in many people, the freak-outs only resurface when stress levels reach a certain point. Unfortunately, for many people, the periods just prior to or soon after a medical procedure are very anxiety-provoking. As a result, the vulnerabilities do resurface but at a time that is too late in the process for the surgeon to take effective remedial steps.

This is why surgeons sometimes find themselves suddenly launched into managing psychological crises at a time when the focus should be on helping a patient either to prepare for a procedure or to heal from one. Even the most caring and compassionate surgeon's office can't be expected to help the patient examine and resolve complex and persistent psychological vulnerabilities, especially in moments of crisis.

An earlier referral for psychotherapy would be much more likely to help the patient. One obvious reason is a mental health professional is trained to provide that kind of treatment. But another benefit of psychotherapy is that its focus is intended to be the psychological issues. A psychotherapy patient comes to the session with the expectation of exploring psychological vulnerabilities. Even a surgeon willing to try to help in this way doesn't have that advantage. It should be noted that even with the expectation of examining psychological functioning, and within the safe confines of the psychotherapy session, prickliness can still be pretty, well, prickly to treat.

Alexis had originally come to me to address the prominent functional deficits to which I alluded earlier. For many years, she had experienced instability in both work and romantic relationships. Also, despite her financial success, she struggled with low self-esteem. There was a mile-wide critical streak running through her. She was lovely, but she was also overly critical of everyone and everything, including herself.

In hindsight, Dr. K said he was aware there were some warning flags he might have picked up on when Alexis first met with him. The problem is, it's often difficult for the surgeon or his staff to know when warning flags are serious enough to warrant a referral to, or consultation with, a psychologist.

One of the first things Alexis revealed to Dr. K was a tendency toward overreactions. Excessive enthusiasm might seem like a form of hopefulness and confidence, but when a new patient exhibits it to an excessive degree, it often foretells a problematic tendency to be too demanding. Put simply, if she placed so much value on Dr. K helping her, it indicates there was a great deal riding on the procedure being successful.

Dr. K might also have noted Alexis's impulsiveness. She presented with a sense of urgency that implied the likelihood of impulse control issues. This is a potential problem given these procedures always require patience during the healing period.

Perhaps the biggest red flags were revealed in Alexis's description of Dr. K's work on her friends. During their initial meeting, Alexis told Dr. K that she believed he had "saved" her friend's face. Alexis also used extreme language to describe her friends' appearances. Dr. K. is human, so it would be understandable for him to have basked in those compliments a bit. But the compliments were a tell that Alexis tended to apply rigid and harsh standards to physical qualities in other people. In this way, Alexis's colorful language revealed a tendency to overreact.

Understanding and Addressing "Prickliness"

Mental health professionals develop the ability to quickly detect the kinds of personal qualities Alexis exhibited. Psychologists listen carefully for telltale signs like the tendency to view the same person as a savior one day and a persecutor the next. In a similar vein, although it's good for a prospective patient to feel eager to meet a well-respected surgeon, emotional intensity is a common quality in a person who tends to embrace unreasonable demands. Demands make dissatisfaction with cosmetic procedures more likely. Alexis is an example of a patient whose high intensity was likely detectable by a careful observer.

There are various reasons why people like Alexis acquire their prickly nature. Trauma is one reason: people who are prickly have often been physically and/or emotionally traumatized. Within the context of trauma treatment and recovery, the prickly behavior pattern is a completely predictable, adaptive, and logical response. Abuse causes people to develop behaviors that discourage closeness. In other words, prickly behavior is self-protective. It keeps people at a safe distance. This is why it's so important to be careful about diagnosing prickliness. Prickliness is often misunderstood and is even sometimes misdiagnosed because it's so easy to focus on the prickly behaviors rather than on the underlying causes of them. We understand and respond to prickliness most effectively when we slow down and step back far enough to view it with compassion, respect, and curiosity.

The value of recognizing these struggles in a patient like Alexis is that it enables the physician to get the patient the help they need to make a successful cosmetic outcome more likely. This is why it's sometimes vital for a surgeon to consult with a mental health professional prior to performing a cosmetic service.

The prickly patient's tendency toward dissatisfaction is particularly important for the physician to understand. Because a prickly person often feels dissatisfied, other people learn to behave as though they are walking on eggshells when they are with them. The prickly person effectively teaches people to feel an ever-present danger of failing them. The problem is worsened by the fact that prickly people don't just have high standards, they have excessively high standards, and their punishments for violating the standards are too severe. They are too easily offended and too rarely satisfied.

Physicians need to understand this. So often I have consulted with a physician who feels exasperated by a prickly patient. The doctor will tell me, "I've done excellent work on that patient, but nothing is ever enough!" What the doctor doesn't realize is the prickly patient habitually creates their own displeasure. Usually, the doctor never had a chance.

The patient's powerful agenda is not entirely conscious or voluntary. This may sound strange but it's involuntary in the sense that it becomes a behavioral form of muscle memory. It's reactive. The person reacts in the ways they have practiced. At a certain point, ways of relating to other people become automatic.

Sadly, prickly patients continually create opportunities to feel disappointment. The feeling serves several self-sabotaging functions at once: it maintains distance from the doctor, preserves their dissatisfaction with their own appearance, and reinforces their belief that everything and everyone will fail them.

In case the description above sounds harsh, I want to clarify that I don't intend it to sound rejecting. And I certainly don't intend to encourage you to behave in rejecting ways toward these people—or yourselves. As a psychologist, I happen to like working with prickly people. In my experience, effective psychotherapy typically helps these people learn how to make a more trusting, loving, and less defensive kind of contact with other people. Once they feel safe, they are generally extraordinarily kind, well-intentioned, and compassionate. One key to helping these people is to see and respect their pain. I've never met a prickly person who didn't have good reasons for their prickliness. The ongoing work in psychotherapy is characterized by a collaborative effort to see the real and understandable sadness, fear, anger, and resentment that lie behind the thorns.

Finding Prickers: The P Test

Psychological assessment is a tricky and complicated business. To distinguish exactly what formal diagnosis fits a particular client best, psychologists often utilize a variety of assessment tools. Formal assessments undergo rigorous psychometric validation processes. It's a big deal to attach a psychiatric diagnosis to a person, so before we do that, we exercise great care.

The same level of care is not needed for a screening tool. This kind of tool can be used as a rough indicator that a diagnosable psychological condition might underlie certain behaviors. Prospective patients might benefit from using such a tool on themselves. Likewise, a surgeon might ask a patient to complete a screening tool during the process of considering treating the patient. The P Test (for prickliness) is that kind of a tool. It is a simple, brief measure of emotional wellness. It focuses on sources of emotional vulnerability that are particularly relevant to cosmetic procedures and that a patient would likely benefit from discussing with a mental health professional.

In this book, I've included four simple screening tools that any patient or medical professional can use to identify psychological issues that could undermine the cosmetic outcome. In their own ways, the Appearance Self-Consciousness Measure (ASM), the Body Image Concerns (BIC) Screener, and the MIRROR Test all help a patient assess their tendency to have intense feelings, thoughts, and behaviors related to their perceptions of the way they look and the way they think other people evaluate them.

Now I want to add the P Test. Before presenting this tool, I want to set the proper context for its use. First, this tool should be used to help a person address their needs, not to judge or condemn them. We all struggle. Please try to remember that. The struggles of life give rise to particular needs—in all of us. With the right help, the needs can be diminished and managed. Second, this is a simple screening tool. It should absolutely not be used to diagnose or to draw any firm conclusion about a person's psychological health.

 The P Test

Directions: The questions below call for either a "yes" or "no" response. They ask you to identify general but personal details about how you tend to think, feel, and behave. Your honest responses will help us to better see and address your needs.

1. I get into frequent disagreements with the people closest to me, including friends.

2. People tend to "walk on eggshells" around me.

3. It's not unusual for me to be moody.

4. I often just do things I want to without thinking about consequences.

5. I have caused myself physical pain intentionally, such as by cutting, scratching, biting, or burning myself.

6. I have struggled with suicidal thoughts at times in my life.

7. I often feel like people can't be trusted.

8. I have felt abandoned sometimes by close friends or family members.

9. I tend to become consumed in things (eating, gaming, smoking, drinking, exercise, sex, shopping, etc.).

10. I go through periods when I really don't like myself.

11. Sometimes I feel powerless to communicate how I really feel.

12. People often fail me.

13. I have abused substances in the past.

Scoring. Even a single "yes" response to any of the items is likely a helpful subject for some exploration in psychotherapy prior to undergoing a cosmetic procedure. Three or more "yes" responses should certainly be considered a red flag, indicating that the patient is more likely than most to struggle with the uncertainty and subjectivity of a cosmetic procedure outcome. Consultations with mental health professionals would likely be helpful during such a patient's course of treatment.

The main thrust of this chapter has been that it's especially import-ant for more psychologically vulnerable patients to prepare themselves properly prior to undergoing a cosmetic service. There is no doubt that a successful cosmetic procedure can help a person feel better about the way they look, and this might very well help a person feel better in general. However, it's important to remember that physical changes alone are unlikely to heal chronic and severe psychological distress. Lasting changes in how we think, feel, and behave require focused efforts sustained over time. In other words, we change the inside by starting with the inside, not the outside.

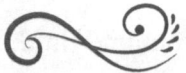

CHAPTER 11

Gem Hunting: Finding the Right Medical Team

The only way in which anyone can lead us is to restore to us the belief in our own guidance.

— *Henry Miller*

The Right Fit

Eric was a forty-year-old attorney. He was vacationing with his wife, outside of the United States. While his wife was getting a facial at the Olivia & Hemmingway Beauty Spa, Eric sat and perused the menu of services. He sipped the perfect cappuccino the receptionist made for him with the on-site Italian espresso machine.

As Eric admired the menu's beautiful design, an attendant approached and began chatting with him about the services. He indicated he was there only because his wife was receiving a service and that he was not interested in any service.

A friendly conversation ensued. Mainly, they focused on the sourcing of the delicious coffee. The subject did, however, return to the cosmetic services on offer. Eric acknowledged that he and his wife had noticed that the prices were significantly lower than what they would find at home. Impulsively, Eric decided to undergo a Botox treatment to eliminate forehead wrinkles. As is typical of Botox treatments, it was fast and relatively painless.

Soon after the treatment, Eric noticed his eyebrows were sitting unusually low on his forehead. He consulted with a physician after returning home and learned that the person administering the Botox created this problem; the Botox should have been administered differently. Fortunately, Eric's eyebrow problem would likely be temporary.

The lesson Eric learned was that even common cosmetic services are not without risk. Like other medical procedures, success requires a skillful professional, the right procedure, and an appropriately equipped location.

This chapter is devoted to the process of choosing the right surgeon and facility. I intend in this chapter to speak not only to patients, but also to surgeons and their staffs. It's important for medical professionals to be aware of the very real difficulties prospective patients encounter in the process of finding a surgical team that feels like the right fit. Cosmetic surgery patients often have particular needs. It's best if both the patients and physicians are sensitized to that and address the needs openly, directly, and compassionately.

Qualifications of Surgeons

When looking for a surgeon who possesses the ideal combination of training, skills, and experience, the patient can start with the formal standards to which physicians are held in the community where the procedure will occur. Standards are typically articulated by the appropriate licensing agencies in that location. In the United States, licensure is managed at the state level. Every state has a board that determines the criteria for licensure that surgeons must meet.

If you are considering a location outside the United States, you will likely consult that nation's national licensing body—but perhaps not. The standards for licensure in a given country may be determined by a national board, or they may resemble the United States and have licensure guided by regional boards. It's very important that you find physicians who are licensed, but it's equally important that you seek independent information regarding the local licensure standards where a prospective surgeon is located.

In addition to local licensure guidelines, patients should also learn about the standards embraced by the leading regulating medical associations. Many years ago, a surgeon was a surgeon. The same surgeon who performed facial procedures would perform procedures on other parts of the body. In that earlier time, there were no formal training programs for surgeons after medical school. Nowadays, surgeons often specialize not only in cosmetic work but often only in particular types of cosmetic procedures.

This means patients can be very selective and well-informed about their surgeon's qualifications and experience. Patients who do their research can learn about the standards set forth by the leading surgeons in the relevant areas of medicine. Patients can then examine the degree to which the surgical team they are considering meets the highest standards.

Your research may be compromised if you plan to undergo a procedure in a nation with fewer resources. In some locations in the world, it may be much more difficult to find specific and relevant standards set forth by that nation's leading cosmetic surgeons. But you can still protect yourself. If you plan to save money by seeking a procedure in a nation where medical care and skilled nursing assistance are more affordable, you still can—and should—familiarize yourself with the standards that guide treatment when performed in a world-class facility and by a world-renowned surgeon. Once you do that research, you can formulate questions that you bring to the surgical team you are considering. This is one method you can use to assess your comfort level with that team and location.

Licensure, Board Certification, and Fellowship Training

In the United States, the fundamental standard for any physician is the licensing provided by that state's medical board, sometimes called a board of medical examiners. A doctor's licensure status (which shows status, any suspensions, and other practice-related issues) is easily accessible via an online search. The Federation of State Medical Boards has an online site devoted to providing contact information for every state board that licenses doctors in the United States.

In addition to state boards, there are specialty boards that certify physicians for particular specialties. The American Board of Medical Specialties (ABMS) is a nationally recognized not-for-profit organization that "serves the public and the medical profession by improving the quality of health care…in partnership with its twenty-four certifying Member Boards," according to its website (located at www.abms.org at the time of printing). Board certification is intended to inform the public which physicians have distinguished themselves by virtue of their education, knowledge, experience, skills, and commitment to ongoing education. Board-certified surgeons are often referred to as "diplomats" in their specialty area.

Patients sometimes misunderstand the meaning of certain terms when trying to assess a surgeon's qualifications. One source of confusion is that *board-certified* sounds a lot like *fully licensed*. These terms mean very different things. All practicing surgeons in the United States must be licensed. The same would be true of surgeons in other developed nations. In the United States, board certification refers to a higher distinction. A board-certified surgeon has completed more specialized training and experience than an uncertified surgeon. Board certification is some-times referred to as the gold standard because it separates surgeons with advanced specialized training from those who are licensed but are not board-certified.

Another confusing issue is the way physicians often describe their certification status. Terms such as board eligible, board qualified, or board admissible are not the same as board-*certified*. Board-certified indicates the surgeon has already met all of the training, testing, and experience required for certification.

Board certification is intended to provide an objective way patients can compare surgeons' training and experience. Unfortunately, there is yet another complicating factor: there are multiple certifying boards and those boards sometimes compete with one another for member surgeons. Each board seeks to convince consumers that the most skilled surgeons possess their certification as opposed to another organization's certification.

The competition among certifying bodies is readily observable online. For instance, some plastic surgeons who are board-certified by the American Board of Plastic Surgery (ABPS) note on their websites that the ABPS is the only plastic surgery board recognized by the American Board of Medical Specialties. Plastic surgeons' websites sometimes get very specific, expressing the view that the American Board of Facial Plastic and Reconstructive Surgery (ABFPRS) and the American Board of Cosmetic Surgery both offer inferior certifications, as compared to that provided by the ABPS. At the time of this book's printing, one such website expresses the view that ABFPRS certification involves too little focus on general plastic surgery training.

There are, in turn, online sources of information that articulate a different view. Some criticize the political power possessed by the ABPS. Surgeons who are not certified as plastic surgeons sometimes contend that ABPS certification provides preparation that is best suited for reconstructive procedures, as opposed to purely cosmetic ones. Physicians who hold this view believe surgeons certified in general plastic surgery lack the training necessary to make the fine aesthetic alterations that are often required to achieve a successful outcome in an elective procedure that is purely cosmetic. An example of this might be a surgeon who focuses on facial plastic surgery. Oculofacial plastic surgeons, for instance, perform many procedures that they contend require specialized knowledge and training in both ophthalmology and cosmetic surgery. This highly specialized branch of ophthalmology focuses on surgery of the eyelids, eyebrows, tear ducts, and orbit. Oculofacial plastic surgeons often claim that the eye has a particular physiology that can only be understood after years of specialized education including extensive supervised oculofacial plastic surgical training, which general plastic surgeons do not possess.

Another example of boards disagreeing over the skill level of their respective certified members is evident in a recent online article published by the American Society of Plastic Surgeons (ASPS).[6] The article contends that surgeons often perform cosmetic procedures with inadequate preparation. It reports the finding that doctors who advertise themselves as certified by the American Board of Cosmetic Surgery (ABCS) don't measure up to the criteria required of board-certified plastic surgeons.

---

6 Why a "Board-Certified Cosmetic Surgeon" Isn't a Plastic Surgeon, and What That Means for You: Many doctors marketing themselves as cosmetic surgeons do procedures beyond the scope of their training. American Society of Plastic Surgeons website, 10/26/2020 (https://www.plasticsurgery.org/news/press-releases/why-a-board-certified-cosmetic-surgeon-isnt-a-plastic-surgeon-and-what-that-means-for-you).

The article cites a study published in the November 2020 official medical journal of the American Society of Plastic Surgeons (ASPS). In that study, a team led by Brian C. Drolet, MD, of the Vanderbilt University Medical Center reviewed online information to assess residency training history and advertised scopes of practice for 342 ABCS-certified physicians. The study found that 62.6% of ABCS diplomates advertised that they performed surgical procedures that these authors considered to be beyond the advertising physicians' scope of training. The study went so far as to specifically identify the procedures most commonly performed by physicians who lacked the necessary specialized training, as well as the prevalence of incidents of inadequately prepared surgeons performing the procedures. The procedures identified, in order of prevalence, were liposuction (59.6%), abdominoplasty (50.0%), breast augmentation (49.7%), and buttock augmentation (36.5%).

So, there are some turf wars among competing certifying medical boards. Unfortunately, it's difficult for a nonphysician to intelligently weigh the various perspectives. This is why a consultation with a physician who does not have a vested interest in your choice of surgeon can be especially helpful. Suzanne, a patient who will be discussed later in this chapter, utilized this method.

Beyond board certification, patients can examine a surgeon's training. Some physicians have more specialized advanced training in the form of fellowships than other surgeons. For instance, a patient seeking a liposuction procedure might seek a general plastic surgeon who is board-certified in plastic surgery. Although that would be a reasonably well-informed, intelligent decision, some might contend that, for liposuction procedures involving the face, craniofacial fellowship training would be helpful, as it provides focused training in facial plastic surgery.

In discussing board certification, it's important to note that there are highly skilled surgeons who are not board-certified. Board certification and fellowships are helpful indicators of advanced and specialized training, but it's important to always remember that there are no guarantees. This is why it's so important to adopt a method of finding your surgeon that integrates multiple factors. Some of those factors would be quality of medical school, licensure status, type of residency training, board certification, number and types of fellowships completed, recommendations by past patients, recommendations by physicians in the field, and your own assessment of the degree to which the physician's past patients' before-and-after photos reflect successful examples of the aesthetic goals you seek to achieve.

A Little Help from Your Friends

Caroline was a sixty-three-year-old woman seeking a deep facial peel. Deep facial peels are complex cosmetic interventions that require some anesthesia to minimize patient discomfort. In choosing a surgeon with an appropriate type of board certification for this particular procedure, Caroline might have sought a surgeon board-certified either in plastic surgery or in dermatology. If, however, Caroline had wanted a peel that would firm up the skin underneath her eyes, she might have sought a surgeon board-certified in ophthalmology.

So, Caroline had a difficult decision to make in choosing the right kind of surgeon—even once she narrowed her search down to specialist surgeons. This is because board-certified plastic surgeons sometimes subspecialize in, say, "surgery of the hand" or in "plastic surgery within the head and neck." So, perhaps Caroline should only have sought a surgeon with a particular subspecialty certification.

Caroline's task was difficult, but not impossible. To do it well would require an investment in both time and effort. Caroline would have to conduct some research. If she could speak briefly with a few physicians who do not perform facial peels but who have expertise in plastic surgery, ophthalmology, or dermatology, she would probably acquire some very helpful guidance. A physician who does not do peels may be more likely to offer unbiased information because they would have no personal stake in the advice. The problem is they might not offer the consultation if they don't do peels. Caroline could also do some online research, being careful to choose only sources that have verifiably informed viewpoints.

Let's now turn to an example of a patient who was able to succeed in using the available information to make informed decisions about her treatment. Suzanne, a sixty-two-year-old financial planner, intended to undergo an eyelid procedure. Suzanne began her process by consulting her own ophthalmologist, Dr. G, who approved of Suzanne's decision to undergo the elective cosmetic work. Since Dr. G does not provide that particular service but is an ophthalmologist, Suzanne considered Dr. G to be a trustworthy source for reliable, nonbiased, expert information and advice. Suzanne asked Dr. G: "How would you choose a surgeon if you were me?" Dr. G told Suzanne that, generally, the most important board certification for a cosmetic surgeon operating on a patient's eyes is ophthalmology. Dr. G then directed Suzanne to online cosmetic surgery referral sources where Suzanne could search among many surgeons.

Suzanne found three surgeons through online research. In her initial search, she looked for surgeons who had graduated from well-regarded medical schools and who had completed fellowships—the more the better, so long as the training involved cosmetic work or eye surgeries.

All three of Suzanne's finalists were board-certified. One of them was not certified in ophthalmology, so Suzanne eliminated that one. Suzanne then asked Dr. G whether she knew either of the two oculofacial plastic surgeons on her list. Dr. G immediately indicated that Dr. X, one of the two, was well-regarded and did consistently excellent work. Dr. X also tended to produce subtle cosmetic outcomes, which was another of

Suzanne's preferences. Suzanne chose Dr. X, and she was very happy with the result.

One of the most important lessons to take from Suzanne's example is that your own physicians can be great resources in your search for the right procedure and cosmetic surgeon. In Dr. G, Suzanne found a physician who knew Suzanne's condition, knew a great deal about oculofacial plastic surgery, and was familiar with the work of various cosmetic surgeons. After all, Dr. G sees surgical outcomes frequently and in fine detail, often looking at eyes through special magnifying devices.

Suzanne's approach can be generalized to other types of procedures. For instance, an ear, nose, and throat doctor who does not do cosmetic work might be a great resource for a patient seeking a skilled surgeon to perform a cosmetic procedure on some part of the face. A patient's dermatologist might be of assistance in the same way, if the dermatologist does not perform the desired procedure. A physician who specializes in gastrointestinal disorders might know of surgeons who are skilled in tummy tucks, liposuction, or other similar procedures.

Professional Societies

Another resource patients might consider in choosing a physician is membership in a professional society. These organizations limit memberships in various ways, often to certain types of specialists. Some societies only admit physicians who have demonstrated superior skills.

Prospective patients can find out which professional organizations exist and what the standards are for membership. Patients might also learn which societies create and monitor standards of practice within the given specialty. The American Society of Plastic Surgeons (ASPS) is one such organization, and the California Society of Plastic Surgeons is another. The ASPS website (www.plasticsurgery.org) provides a wonderful discussion of the various ways a patient might assess a cosmetic surgeon under consideration. In looking over the ASPS suggestions, the subjectivity of the process becomes clear: no physician is the single best choice for every patient. There is an indescribable "fit" component unique to each doctor-patient relationship. The ASPS website offers a wealth of helpful suggestions for assessing the fit between you and the physicians you are considering.

Before leaving the subject of board certification and membership in professional societies, let's briefly discuss bureaucracies. It's good to be mindful that these are all bureaucratic organizations. As with any large organization, politics influences the ways professional boards and societies qualify and grant special recognition to certain members of their profession. It's important to remain mindful that physicians differ in their views regarding what training and experiences are necessary to become highly skilled in a particular cosmetic surgical procedure. This is yet another reason it can be helpful to consult with a physician who has knowledge of the given topic but no vested interest in the opinion they express to you.

Bedside Manner

Melinda felt conflicted. She had met with Dr. Y once before. Today, she met with him again. Dr. Y had been recommended by her internist, whom Melinda likes very much. About her latest meeting with Dr. Y, Melinda explained, "I don't dislike Dr. Y, I just feel like he is disinterested in me. After our most recent consultation, I commented that I like the color he chose for the walls in the waiting room. I added that you don't often see that color of rose in medical settings. He half-smiled, closed the manila file holding my medical record, and turned and walked out. And that was it. He left. No 'good-bye,' no 'thank you,' no 'nice to have seen you.' He just left. I just feel no connection with him."

As a seventy-one-year-old woman who was meeting with Dr. Y to explore undergoing facial plastic surgery, Melinda's experience provides us with an example of something we already know: physicians have personalities and, like all of us, their personalities tend to fit better with some people than they do with others. It's important that plastic surgery patients consider the fit between their personality and the personality of the physician under consideration.

Every patient wants to get along with their doctor, but within the plastic surgery context, this issue often carries greater relevance. Plastic surgery patients have more of a need to communicate openly about sensitive topics with their doctor. For example, a patient who has struggled with anxiety will likely want to find a doctor capable of remaining patient and sensitive while addressing concerns and uncertainties.

Fortunately, many cosmetic surgeons respond with compassion to the psychological vulnerabilities of their patients. The most skilled surgeons discuss risk-related matters in ways that invite open dialogue and questions. This often helps the patient feel reassured, while the physician gains a preview of how the patient tends to respond to reassurance and cope with ambiguity and risk. I have found physicians skilled in assessing their patients' mental health use these discussions to inform their decision to refer an emotionally vulnerable patient to a psychologist who can help prepare the patient for the surgery process.

Psychological vulnerabilities can reveal themselves in a variety of ways. A patient who has undergone past cosmetic procedures may bring a particular set of expectations for emotional support from the physician. Patients who intend to travel a great distance for a procedure to a place far away from their home, family, and friends have their own reasons for perhaps needing extra support. When planning to undergo a procedure without the benefit of family and friends being near, they may consider it even more important that communications with the doctor be open, clear, and encouraged.

Another reason patients often prioritize finding a doctor who *feels* supportive is the vulnerability experienced during the recovery period. Postsurgical monitoring is vitally important to confirm healthy healing. Every patient needs to communicate with their surgeon about this during the recovery period. Assessing healing, typically within the context of some degree of physical limitation and discomfort, gives rise to feelings of vulnerability. Even under the best of circumstances, during the monitoring and healing process, open and supportive communication with the surgeon is not only important medically, but also for nurturing a healing mindset in the patient.

The physician and the patient both have personality characteristics that are discernible in the initial consultations. It's good for all involved to be observant of these characteristics, no matter how brief the meetings. Certain questions might seem to upset the surgeon or their staff members. The physician's response may discourage more questions. For example, a surgeon may seem defensive when asked why they chose their particular board certification over a different certification and what relevance the surgeon's choice might have for this patient's planned procedure. That would be a smart question for a patient to ask. If the surgeon were to respond in a prickly way, it would be fair for the patient to factor that into their assessment of the physician's openness. It's vitally important, for both the patient and the doctor, that the patient not feel the need to refrain from asking questions.

While there should be room in the discussion to address the patient's concerns, the questions should be reasonable and should be asked respectfully. Just as the patient will want to carefully observe, it's also prudent for the physician to notice client attitudes that may foreshadow excessive demands and rigidity.

The bottom line? The initial discussions are difficult and the difficulties may provide important information about whether the fit between the patient and physician is good enough. Sometimes it simply isn't. And there isn't always a person who is obviously at fault. Think of it this way: anytime people engage in a discussion, the people can be thought of like chemicals. When chemicals are combined, they create a chemical compound. So, any discussion is like a chemical compound. Both the surgeon and the patient benefit by carefully assessing whether their compound seems too flammable or explosive. Sometimes, the best way to avoid explosions is to keep the chemicals apart, by the patient finding a different doctor.

Patients can enhance their assessment of these issues by bringing a relative or friend to the consultation. The friend can be tasked with asking the tougher questions. Regardless of who asks the questions, after the meeting the patient should ask the friend to share their impressions. This helps the patient evaluate whether this physician is the right one, given this patient's needs.

Artistic Sensibilities

In choosing their surgeon, cosmetic surgery patients often try to assess the physician's artistry. Cosmetic surgeons frequently encourage this by expressing the view that the doctor's artistic sensibility plays a central role in the success of the procedure. This idea is commonly reinforced indirectly by the meticulous care many cosmetic surgeons show in making design choices that are on display in their offices, on their websites, and in any promotional material they produce for public consumption.

Perhaps the most relevant way in which the surgeon's aesthetic vision is revealed is in before-and-after photographs. Those photographs provide impressions of what that physician considered to be successful outcomes. Patients can use these photos to determine whether they share compatible definitions of beauty with the physician. One specific example of this involves patients' tendency to choose surgeons whose outcomes appear to be natural.

On the one hand, the patient's sense of the surgeon's aesthetic can help patients to make prudent choices. However, these gross markers should not replace careful discussions with the surgeon. For instance, design choices in the physician's physical office space can be misleading because they might say more about the surgeon's ability to find a talented interior decorator than they say about the surgeon's artistry in the operating room. This may also be true of the physician's website and other marketing materials. Likewise, surgeons might carefully sift through before-and-after photos to choose the ones that present their skill level in ways that don't reflect the reality.

Patient Reviews

It's not uncommon for physicians to receive online reviews. Prospective patients often look online for reviews written by past patients of the doctor being considered. This approach is often criticized. Some people might suggest that other issues, such as the surgeon's training and certification status, should be considered more important. Still others contend that the focus should be on the consultation and the patient's own impressions of the doctor during it.

Problems can arise when patients rely solely on patient reviews. Reviews are sometimes overly influenced by details that are more important to the reviewer than they would be to other people. And significant details are sometimes not mentioned. For instance, an overly critical review might fail to reveal that the surgical procedure involved an unusual degree of complexity due to the reviewer's physical condition at the time. Similarly, a dissatisfied reviewer might also not be transparent about their own tendency to rarely feel satisfied.

One strategy to improve the usefulness of online reviews is to search for objective information in them. Descriptions of facilities and services can often be provided in objective ways. It's true that ratings of a facility's decorative and design choices may be subjective, but a careful prospective patient can often separate out the facts to obtain objective data.

Distinguishing between subjective and objective review comments can be tricky. Subjectivity is often couched within objective information and vice versa. Here is a hypothetical review that illustrates the issue:

> "During my recovery, I felt abandoned constantly. My nurse had too many other patients. And the single nurse's aid who was assigned to my nurse never allowed me to sleep! Whenever I complained, he or my nurse blamed the facility's procedures, saying they were required to check my bandages or my swelling or document data in my record and that there was a rigid schedule requiring each. And yet, when I specifically asked for an alternative to plastic eating utensils, I never got any help. The aide kept insisting he could not find me a single metal fork and knife. Really?!! In the entire facility? Ridiculous. Those are examples of the poor staffing and services at this facility."

This imaginary review contains some helpful information that the subjective elements might hide from view. In terms of subjective aspects of the review, the patient seems difficult to please. It's helpful to recognize that an overly demanding patient is more likely to feel dissatisfied. A related issue to consider is that unpleasant patients might unfortunately receive less attentive care because the nursing staff might want to avoid interacting with them. Although avoidance is not a good way for nurses to manage a prickly patient, this does suggest a different patient might receive better care. So, certain aspects of this review would likely not be helpful to the general reader.

Despite this reviewer's biases, this review does provide some useful objective information about the facility. For instance, on the plus side, the staff at the facility seem to be attentive to standards and protocols related to direct patient care. Those practices protect the patient and that's important information for a prospective patient to have. In fact, the reviewer's own descriptions of staff behaviors seem to cast doubt on the accusation of understaffing.

Second Opinions

As you search for information about physicians, try to be mindful of the potential impact of bias. You can certainly expect reputable physicians and their staff to be truthful. Still, there is truth and there is truth.

Joseph, a thirty-eight-year-old accountant who believed he needed a procedure to remove under-eye bags, consulted an oculofacial specialist to explore undergoing a lower blepharoplasty. The surgeon examined Joseph, and they discussed pricing and scheduling. Joseph then went to another oculofacial surgeon to discuss the same procedure and compare prices and practices. The second surgeon said she would not perform that operation on Joseph because his condition warranted only a minor injection of filler. Joseph decided the second surgeon was acting more in Joseph's interests and he chose the minor filler procedure.

The point of retelling Joseph's story is not to suggest that the first surgeon was unethical and was intentionally recommending a procedure Joseph didn't need. Although that might have been the case, I suspect this was more likely a matter of two surgeons arriving at different conclusions. That happens all the time. There are normally multiple ways to achieve a cosmetic change. It's left to the patient to consult with surgeons and discuss each surgeon's suggestions carefully to assess which recommended course of action best achieves the patient's objectives.

The patient needs to exercise due diligence. Second opinions are recommended because they help the prospective patient continue to explore their unique set of needs and preferences. Physicians who seem to discourage second opinions should be considered with heightened caution.

Conflicts of Interest Impacting Your Search for Important Information

Ideally, patients should know all relevant details before choosing to undergo a surgical procedure. One reason it can be difficult to find all of the information is that not all of it has equal relevance for all patients. The physicians don't always know what a particular prospective patient needs to know.

Another reason a patient might not obtain all of the important information prior to undergoing a procedure is that it isn't always communicated in a way that effectively informs the patient. This may be due to communication difficulties. Sometimes, however, cosmetic patients report to me that they believed the physician's office intentionally left certain details out when the procedure was scheduled. Fairly or unfairly, those patients told me they believed bias was the reason they didn't obtain all of the important information prior to the procedure.

Bias can show up in various ways. One common source of bias is conflict of interest. There is an unavoidable reality that a medical practice has a financial interest in performing medical services. That reality causes some patients to be suspicious of physicians' recommendations.

In my experience, although it's good for patients to exercise due diligence, I don't believe patients should expect to be sold and upsold various cosmetic procedures. I think much of the time the problem arises in more subtle ways than intentional upselling. For instance, unfortunately, personnel in a physician's office might inadvertently fail to inform patients about every important aspect of the surgery and recovery process. At the same time, patients often understandably don't know what they don't know, and so they fail to ask the particular questions that would address their unique situation.

Paul's case is a good one to discuss on this subject because he was unhappy with aspects of his experience, and while it's not entirely clear that bias played a role in his problems, it might have. Paul was a forty-six-year-old male client who underwent a successful and yet somewhat disastrous liposuction procedure on his torso. The procedure occurred in the middle of June. You'll soon understand why this was a relevant detail.

Paul is a successful restauranteur. He's a funny, playful guy who is well-liked and likes to be somewhat unpredictable. One of the issues his therapy addressed was his tendency to be a people-pleaser. He also made a habit of relying on his instincts. For instance, once he told me he had the inspiration to offer an "International Pasta Pocket Night." The special meal began with a Polish pierogi appetizer, followed by soup with Russian pelmeni, and then an Italian beef ravioli main course, and finished off with a big, sweet-cheese, fried ravioli for dessert. His creativity and impulsiveness were assets to his business. He had a loyal clientele who loved his inspirations.

Paul was also a workaholic who felt frustrated with how his body had changed in recent years. He had long considered a procedure that would eliminate fat such as by freezing it or by using a laser on it. One day, after reading about a liposuction technique, he decided to have the surgical procedure. It was focused on his lower abdomen.

His surgeon had a cancellation, enabling him to bump Paul up on the schedule to a date that was sooner than originally planned. Being somewhat impulsive, Paul was pleased to *not* have a lot of time to think about it.

The procedure went smoothly. From a medical perspective, he was satisfied with the outcome. But he was unhappy for other reasons. I didn't see Paul from the time of the procedure until about ten weeks after it.

When we met and I asked him how it went, he explained, "After the procedure, my recovery was on track. During the checkup two weeks after the lipo, the doc casually informs me that I may need to wear the compression jacket most of the time for another four to six weeks, maybe even until August."

"That surprised you?"

"Of course it surprised me. I had a beach vacation planned for the end of July. I had told him that when we first met. I even spoke about it with his calendar-minder because she asked me which resort I'd chosen."

Then I remembered a detail Paul had shared with me. I said, "Wait a minute. Weren't you going to have the procedure the first week of August?"

"Exactly. Yes. That was the plan. But then he had a cancellation so I got in six weeks sooner. I don't know, maybe he forgot about my vacation because it wouldn't have been an issue if I'd had the lipo in August."

Paul explained that his first problem was his beach vacation. He had no desire to wear a compression jacket on the beach. In addition, his business partner had a vacation planned for the first two weeks of July. So, Paul had agreed to be at the restaurant in early July. When he agreed to move the procedure up, he hadn't factored in these issues.

He explained, "There's no way I could have worn that garment to Cabo. And there was no way I could have worn it to work without my staff knowing I'd had a procedure. Not to mention, do you know how hot that garment is? How could the doc not warn me about that? It'd be impossible to wear it in my restaurant in July. The garment is foam. When I wore it I felt like a big, fat, walking, wet sponge. A good look for a horror movie. A restaurant? Not so much."

"What a predicament," I said. "So, what happened?"

"My wife covered for me. She was pissed but not as pissed as I was at the doc. I mean, I assumed the garment needed to be worn for a week or two. We never really discussed the specifics until *after* the procedure.

That's what really pissed me off. I mean, maybe I should have asked more questions but he's the one who knows what's needed after the lipo. He should have told me. I told him about the Cabo trip planned for mid-July. To be honest, I wonder if these doctors just don't want to lose the summer business because it's a slower time for them. I mean, how could he have not talked about all these details before the procedure? I'd never have done it in June if I'd known."

Paul's experience might have been different if he had brought a friend to his surgical consults. Although some patients are shy and need an assertive friend to accompany them, that wasn't Paul's problem. But Paul needed a friend who could slow down the meeting with the surgeon just enough to be sure these important scheduling issues would be discussed.

Paul isn't alone. Whether due to shyness, fear, intimidation when talking with a surgeon, impulsivity, or some other reason, patients often forget to ask even the most basic questions. This is why it's usually very helpful to bring someone to your consultations. You want the person to be someone who can play whatever role is needed to help you make the best decision given your particular situation.

Before meeting with your surgeon, it's best to discuss your plans and concerns in detail with your friend. Encourage that person to ask you probing questions prior to the meeting with the physician so that both of you have a clear understanding of the issues that need to be addressed with the surgeon. Urge your friend to be ready and able to play an active role so that all important issues get discussed.

When Conflict of Interest Is a Pain

I've had a number of clients report that they thought their doctor downplayed the issue of pain prior to the procedure. Some clients have suggested they thought this happened because the doctor didn't want to scare the patient away and lose the business. If this ever happened, it would be an example of a conflict of interest influencing a physician's behavior.

Let's begin with a true and positive piece of information. In my experience, more often than not, my clients who have undergone cosmetic procedures have reported that the pain they experienced was far less than they feared. Unfortunately, physicians and their staff may point to this and wrongly say this justifies only briefly discussing pain and discomfort with a patient prior to their procedure.

Surgeons should certainly discuss issues such as pain, discomfort, and the likelihood that assistance will be needed in the days after the procedure. Abigail, a forty-three-year-old client, spoke with me about the issue of pain after she had recovered from a procedure. Abigail had an under-eye laser treatment. She explained, "I knew my face would swell. And I knew I would need to moisturize and ice my face after the procedure. And I was expecting to be uncomfortable, even very uncomfortable. But I didn't know what the pain would be like. When I asked the surgeon's assistant, she said it would be manageable and that I needn't worry. It felt like a pat on the head. It was insulting."

Abigail said she found the pain to be far more acute than she expected. "It was two or more times more intense than the worst sunburn I have ever had. What bothers me is I think I would have coped better had I simply been told exactly what to expect. I could have prepared myself for it. I think they intentionally understated the pain and that is just not acceptable."

I found Abigail's description believable, especially because I have had other clients share similar experiences. I suspect at least some physicians are guilty of this to some degree. I assume they do it to avoid the problem of patients overthinking the pain issue and thereby exacerbating the discomfort. This is a valid concern. There is research examining the role our psychology plays in our pain tolerance and it seems clear we can make our pain worse by the way we think about it. For instance, if a patient becomes consumed in fear-based anticipation of pain, that may very well impair their pain tolerance. Still, it's best that patients seeking information be provided accurate and complete responses to their questions.

Rather than neglecting to give accurate information, a physician's office should be transparent. They should simply observe patients' reactions to the information. If a patient seems excessively fearful, the patient should be referred to a mental health professional who is able to help the patient to better manage their pain.

The physician's obligation to inform does not replace the patients' obligations to themselves. Patients need to do their own research in addition to asking questions of the doctor and their staff. Issues such as healing times, best recovery practices, and postsurgical lifestyle limitations are best addressed by a combination of independent research and discussions with various informed individuals, in addition to consulting the physician and staff.

Location, Location, Location—and "Medical Tourism"

Contrary to the real estate maxim, a physician's location may not reflect the quality of the work. There are talented cosmetic surgeons in cities throughout the world. In the United States, for example, patients might expect the best surgeons to be located in large cities. In fact, some board-certified surgeons receive extensive training in great research hospitals located in major cities and then choose to locate their practice outside an urban center. Some of those exceptionally skillful surgeons prefer the lifestyle permitted by a suburban or rural location.

Some patients specifically search for surgeons in remote locations or even in other countries. Cosmetic work in certain countries tends to be lower in cost. The decision to have a medical procedure in another country has become so common, a term has been created for it: medical tourism.

People engage in medical tourism for various reasons. Sometimes it is due to the unavailability of a particular treatment in their home state or country. Some treatments are not legal in certain countries. Or the treatment is not yet available in the patient's home country because it requires advanced training and/or equipment that the location does not yet possess. In still other cases, regulatory standards may make the surgery riskier in the person's home country. Lower licensure standards, less rigorous training, and less required experience can all lead to medical complications.

Perhaps the most common reason for medical tourism is cost. This is especially true when the patient lives in a nation such as the US or the UK. Due to the typical high cost of cosmetic procedures in those countries, patients often undergo the procedure in a nation with lower medical costs such as Poland, Hungary, Mexico, Colombia, or Thailand.

The decision to travel to another country may result from issues other than the cost of the procedure itself. All surgical interventions require a postoperative recovery period. Some surgeries, such as complex cosmetic procedures, require extensive postoperative nursing and other support to prevent infection and maximize the likelihood of achieving optimal results. Optimal care often involves changing bandages, monitoring healing, cleaning wounds, and acquiring assistance with medications. Procedures such as liposuction might also involve specialized types of massage and other care such as hyperbaric oxygen treatments to aid recovery. The costs associated with the healing process lead some patients to choose remote locations where both private nursing and costs of living are lower.

Patients who travel to save money are also often swayed by the existence of fully integrated surgical and recovery centers. For instance, just as hotels and many human services are less costly in certain countries, the patient also often saves money on the cost of recovery centers. These are often conveniently located within or adjacent to the medical center where the surgery is conducted. This convenience is particularly valuable while recovering from a surgical procedure. In addition, some patients prefer to be in another country because it grants them privacy. Being so far from home makes it much less likely an intrusive family member, friend, or gossipy neighbor will learn about the procedure.

Of course, the choice to travel is not without risk. Costs are sometimes lower because certain standards are lower. This is not always true, though, and it is also not necessarily true that surgeons in countries with lower medical costs will be less skilled. For instance, some pioneering surgeons in liposuction techniques are in South American nations that often offer lower procedure and recovery center expenses. It's important to carefully consider all these factors. Any quality deficit, whether in the surgeon, the assisting medical personnel, or the facilities, will tend to raise the likelihood of an undesired surgical outcome.

Gathering Information about the Surgical and Postoperative Facilities

Many people feel powerless to choose the right locations for their surgery and recovery processes. They often have no idea which qualities would make a facility more or less desirable. As a result, they de-emphasize the importance of research into the facilities during the planning phase. This is unfortunate. The truth is, we don't have to be experts in the medical or hospital administration fields to evaluate a facility's quality.

You will find plenty of information online. Gather information from multiple sources. Confirm a facility is in good standing by examining public records available online (look for any past code violations, for instance). Search for lawsuits naming the facility you are considering. And, as mentioned earlier, look through patient reviews.

And always consider the source of the information you have found. Online information often contains bias. We always need to consider the possibility that a source might benefit from creating an inaccurate description. For instance, a physician who owns an adjacent recovery center directly benefits from patients using that center.

Some sources, such as regulatory bodies or public records, are more likely to be independent. This diminishes bias problems. These sources generally reveal helpful information about issues related to building, health, or medical code compliance.

In looking for resources, it's often helpful to prioritize highly regarded, science-based sources of information open to the general public. The National Institutes of Health, the Mayo Clinic, or the American Society of Plastic Surgeons are examples of well-respected public sources of information. Today, nations such as Canada, the United States, and most nations in Europe sponsor efforts to provide detailed quality of care information that is readily accessible to the public. The NHS, for instance, plays an active role in seeking to inform consumers regarding this issue in the United Kingdom. These types of resources are less likely to be as accessible or as informative in countries that offer less costly procedure and recovery options.

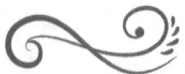

CHAPTER 12

Resilience: Maintaining Emotional Wellness Using Daily Meditations and Affirmations

Meditation practice isn't about trying to throw ourselves away and become something better. It's about befriending who we are already.

— **Pema Chödrön**

Daily Mindfulness

In this chapter you'll find twenty-eight meditations for use during the two weeks prior to and following your cosmetic procedure. They contain affirmations and mantras specifically intended to activate healthy preparations for and recovery from a cosmetic procedure.

Although written with cosmetic services in mind, the meditations speak to issues that arise any time we are seeking support as we grow and change. You might utilize these in a purely meditative process, assisting you to practice mindfulness. Or you might integrate the meditations into an existing or budding formal practice. Use them in whatever ways you find helpful.

The meditations are arranged in a particular chronological order to coincide with certain periods of time prior to or after a surgical procedure. It's best that you commit to the use of these and to the practice of meditation, and that you take ownership of the process. That said, you may want to treat the order of the meditations as a mere guideline, to help you get started. The chronological order isn't intended to be considered a rigid, rule-based formula for success. Like the success of your surgical procedure, the value you find in these meditation tools will depend not on your compliance with a set of rules, but on your commitment to a process characterized by self-compassion and self-care.

This chapter essentially contains twenty-eight meditation tools. Aside from the order in which you read these tools, you may wonder whether you should read them all in one sitting and, if not, how much time you should dedicate to sitting and meditating on the contents of each page. Although I still encourage you to use them in the way that suits your needs, I would suggest reading through them all first and then returning to them to use them as part of your meditation practice.

When using the meditations, some users will prefer to follow a formal schedule of one meditation per day. Others will choose to do more than one per day. Still others will not follow the chronological order at all, preferring instead to select meditations based on what topics feel most relevant on a given day. Those are all perfectly acceptable approaches. To focus on a particular issue one day, you may want to look to the titles to help you distinguish among meditations by subject matter.

Practice Tools

This book is a manual for uncovering a more resilient mindset. In the broadest sense, I hope to help you cope with any of the struggles life sends your way. In this chapter, you will find potent tools that are particularly aimed at developing a sense of empowerment that will assist you during your cosmetic procedure journey.

In the days leading up to the procedure, you will feel more positive and self-supportive if you have nurtured a habit of self-care. The daily meditations in this chapter provide a focused way to do that. They give you an opportunity to stop and dedicate a few moments of each day to the process of preparing for your surgical procedure.

As you examine and use these tools, devote yourself to being mindful. Think of any tool you have—a knife, a screwdriver, or even something as simple as dental floss. Once you pick up dental floss, you explore how you will use that piece of string to help you clean between all your teeth. It probably took a little time to decide exactly how you would use the floss to achieve your goal. You think about how to use the floss because you know that, once you decide how the tool can assist you, the tool becomes more valuable to you.

Try to notice how the tools in this chapter can be used to assist your process. Notice the ways they help you explore the nature of your process. Being mindful in these ways also enhances your commitment to self-care, even if only for minutes per day. Your awareness of your self-care will help you feel more resilient.

Some subjects within the meditations are addressed more than once. However, the specific meditations and quotes on a given page are never repeated in other pages.

The ideas and coping methods are diverse. They expose you to a variety of perspectives but point you in the same direction: toward personal empowerment and self-compassion. These qualities will be the most help-ful ones as you prepare for a cosmetic service. After you recover, if you continue to nurture these same qualities within you, you will experience continued growth and benefits that extend beyond the specific focus of this book.

How to Use these Meditations

Clients unfamiliar with meditation often want specific instructions. That's understandable. Yet one of the functions of a pure mindfulness medita-tion is to practice living less reactively, with more freedom and self-com-passion. In this way, meditation can help a person feel less constrained by rigid demands and rules.

Earlier in the book, I suggested an image for your mindfulness medi-tation. I encouraged you to imagine being a fish surrounded by baited hooks that symbolize your thoughts. I told you to see yourself effortlessly gliding through the water, past the hooks. The objective was to not engage any of the thoughts by biting onto a hook, even though you might want to.

I explained that this type of meditation is designed to give you practice being present with yourself rather than being distracted by your thoughts. The state of distraction is likened to being a fish on a hook; the fish being mercilessly yanked back and forth, in whatever direction the fishing line chooses. The aim of this kind of meditation is to create a space in your mind where there is no yanking. A space where you can practice just "being" rather than constantly reacting and "doing." Ultimately, mind-fulness meditation helps us practice managing the unhealthy tendency to fill our lives with distractions.

I've mentioned that there are many types of meditations. In this chapter, I provide meditations that are different from pure mindfulness meditations. The meditations in this chapter have particular intentions and messages. They are designed to help focus your thoughts and feelings in ways that will help nurture more self-compassion and resilience.

A pure mindfulness meditation asks you to be the fish. As the fish, you try to swim freely, unconstrained by hooks attached to fishing lines. In other words, your goal is to be free of your overly active brain. As you improve, you will notice thoughts but you will neither push them away nor grab at them. You will just coexist peacefully and separately from them, sort of like a neighbor with whom you have a friendly but not close relationship. Neighbors you like enough to be cooperative, but not enough to have over for dinner.

In this chapter, I want you to practice two other kinds of meditation. These meditations both involve intentionally engaging your thoughts, considering them to be tools that improve your life if you take good care of them. So, in these two types of meditations, I want you to treat your thoughts like close personal friends who are there for you when you need support.

I suggest the following approach to the meditations in this chapter. Before reading each page, I recommend beginning with a simple breathing exercise that involves slow, mindful breathing (there is more discussion of breathing techniques later in this chapter). Once you reach a relaxed, focused state, mindfully read the quote and meditation on that page. Take your time reading them. Allow yourself to assess the meaning they have for you.

Each meditation occurs after a quote and a short passage you will find on each page. The meditation will simply involve a moment of sitting, focusing on the quote and the set of ideas presented on the page, beneath the quote. For this brief period, I suggest you sit and allow these ideas to roam around in your mind. Try to notice how they impact you. Allow yourself to indulge these thoughts. See whether the thoughts introduce you to other thoughts that are also friendly and supportive. Be observant.

Next, on each page you will find affirmations and mantras that continue the same theme as the quote and the short passage you just meditated on. Read the affirmations and mantras and then choose a mantra to use as the focal point of another meditation. The mantras are provided to give you a single, empowering idea to focus on during the second meditation for the given page. As you meditate, you may be aware of other thoughts, even friendly ones. The goal is to recognize the other friendly thoughts but continually return your focus to the mantra you chose. This intensifies the impact of the mantra.

There is one more role the mantras play. The mantras can be used the way a gong is used during meditation. Gongs are often used to help people stay present while meditating. A facilitator strikes the gong at random times. The trailing sound of the gong gently reminds participants to bring their wandering mind back into the room.

I suggest you speak the mantra aloud or silently at various times, as if it were a gong. The mantras are brief. You may be able to remember them if you say them a few times to yourself before beginning. Or, you can keep it in front of you so that you can see it at a glance whenever you feel the need to repeat it. Some people do these meditations with their eyes open, to lessen the disruption of glancing and reading while meditating.

The objective of both types of meditations is to help you not only practice staying present, but also engaging in self-care. You will practice activating self-compassion, acceptance, and awareness.

Some clients mistakenly think the goal is to actively problem-solve during these meditations. I don't intend that. I also don't intend you to debate within yourself, such as the idea of whether or not you're too fearful or too concerned about beauty, two of the subjects you will encounter in these pages. Instead of being offered to spur an internal discussion or debate that will help you arrive at a conclusion, the ideas are simply intended to activate whatever thoughts and feelings arise connected to the subject matter.

The goal is to observe the thoughts and feelings that arise within you. To do this, you can borrow from the "wise friend" exercise discussed earlier in this book. Imagine there is a friend within you who is coaching you, encouraging you to simply remain present and aware. Imagine this person is observing you nonjudgmentally during the meditation, encouraging you to remain curious and present with the ideas.

If you'd like, after either meditation you can continue to process your thoughts and feelings by journaling about them. It's best to do this right after completing either or both meditative periods on the page. If you are seeing a therapist, you might consider discussing your journal entries during therapy sessions.

Meditation Location, Comfort, and Setting

The location or "setting" where you choose to meditate is an important decision. People often choose a quiet, private space. Privacy enhances a person's sense of emotional comfort and is helpful when learning a difficult new skill.

But sometimes people choose places for meditation that are loud and full of distractions. Although such a place might feel less safe, comfortable, and quiet, sometimes that's exactly what a person is looking for. People may choose to meditate in a setting that challenges their need for comfort. Since the world isn't always comfortable, and since meditation helps us cope with life's struggles, this can provide valuable practice.

Like the choice of location, the level of physical comfort you choose and how you create that level during your meditation is entirely up to you. There are standing, sitting, and walking meditations. Some people even lie down while meditating. If you sit, you might choose a cushion on the floor, a soft sofa, or a firm chair. Meditation while lying down can be done on any surface, even a hammock.

People who choose to sit rather than lie down often do so to enhance alertness. For this purpose, it helps to maintain an upright but not overly rigid position. You can do this by imagining a string connecting your spine to the ceiling and by holding your chin in a way that keeps your jaw parallel to the floor.

Remember that underlying the mindfulness meditation practice is a commitment to self-compassion. So, if you're working on remaining alert during the meditation, go ahead and take steps to do that, but notice how you are treating yourself in the process. Try to notice if you are being unkind toward yourself when you notice yourself losing alertness. Be curious about your attitude toward yourself. Over time, you will learn more about your body and mind and you will likely improve on your ability to remain alert.

Another aspect of a comfortable setting involves sounds. You may want to listen to some guided meditations. They are easy to find online, such as on YouTube. You might also choose instrumental music.

Breathing While Meditating

When I think about breathing guidelines while meditating, I'm reminded of a line from the great movie Harold and Maude: "How the world dearly loves a cage." Like other areas of our lives, meditation practices can become hijacked by rules. This happens sometimes on the subject of breathing.

Meditation can be a place of refuge from rules. I would humbly suggest it should be, if it is to achieve its most beneficial purpose: mindfulness. Rigid rules about how long to inhale and exhale can cause a counterproductive distraction from mindfulness, even though, ironically, the focus on one's breathing is usually encouraged to aid the meditator to remain present.

The bottom line is that the number of beats you count for each inhalation and exhalation, if you choose to count, depends entirely on your comfort. For most people, it is more relaxing to exhale longer than they inhale. The same is true of holding your breath for a beat or two just after the inhale and before the nice, long, slow exhale. Whatever you do, try to avoid rigid adherence to rules. The key is simply to slow yourself down and practice just being. Use your breath and posture to facilitate those objectives.

Time

There is a giant elephant roaming around these pages: time. This issue touches on how long and how frequently you should meditate. It also involves how many days you should devote to a meditation practice each week, and how long prior to your procedure and how long after the procedure you should meditate.

To establish a regular practice, I recommend beginning with meditations at least five days each week. This may sound like a lot, but the meditations themselves can be brief. Even a single meditation that lasts two or three minutes can suffice in the initial weeks, to get you started. You may find this method will eventually lead you to meditate multiple times in a day. Clients often report this to me.

I want to emphasize that we should avoid claims that sound like prescriptions. Some people who practice meditation will meditate longer than others. That said, I would expect you to benefit most if you eventually increase the meditation time to ten minutes or more, according to your tolerance level. The key is to choose a practice that both fits your tolerance and assists your process of developing a regular meditation practice. Some people might increase their time by doing two or three meditations of two minutes each in a single day, rather than one longer meditation. If you are doing a two-minute meditation, you can even do it in a parking lot, just after or prior to driving. You could also meditate while in a bathroom stall, if need be.

One exception to the no rules advice would be this: don't multitask when you meditate. You will slip into multitasking anyway. We all do. Our minds wander. You will help yourself minimize this if you set the formal intention not to multitask. While you meditate, allow the meditation to be the only thing you do.

Mantras

I've mentioned mantras a number of times. While known in Eastern religions as a sacred phrase repeated over and over, I define mantras as simple, brief phrases repeated to yourself during a meditation, hike, breathing exercise, or some other activity. These phrases are positive, truthful statements we use to remind ourselves of a particular, healthy way of thinking and being. "One step at a time," "I feel grateful," and "I am striving" are examples.

Mantras can be used in various ways. I have found that mantras can dramatically improve a person's self-talk—what we say to ourselves. They can help a person learn how to engage in self-care.

Some people resist mantras, believing them to be unnecessary. Some say that, by stating obvious notions, they feel silly and disempowered when they use them. What those people don't realize is even obvious notions are often blocked from our view, particularly in moments of stress.

To be more specific, mantras are helpful because our self-talk is typically not as self-affirming as it can be. In fact, self-talk is often marked by self-doubt and unkindness. When this happens, our mind fills with judgmental thoughts. In times of stress, the ideas that surge into our conscious mind are the ones we have been feeding our subconscious mind. This is why people often respond with self-criticism in times of stress. Our habitual focus on fears and other overly defensive feelings and thoughts cloud our perceptions, causing us to forget our strengths. This is why mantras serve a corrective function. Mantras provide an empowering message that counters the destructive ones with which we so often fill our minds.

In this chapter, you will see many examples of mantras. Use those that feel helpful to you. It may sound strange for me to suggest that some of mine might not be helpful to you, but it's true. Mantras are personal. I hope those I wrote will speak to you, but the most impactful mantras are often the ones we create for ourselves. So, feel free to do that whenever you'd like. You could also shorten the ones I offer or lengthen them. You will know when you find a good mantra because you will instantly feel the sense of support and nurturance flow within you when you say it to yourself.

Affirmations

Affirmations take various forms. I intend my affirmations to be similar to mantras, but with more detail. I suggest using affirmations to reinforce or affirm inner strength. Like mantras, affirmations work best when they focus on identifying personal strengths and resources as opposed to focusing on deficits. For example, "I approve of myself and see my strengths" would be a better affirmation than "I'm really not such a terrible person." Some other examples of strengths-based messaging to one's self are the following: "I know that I have kind intentions," "I affirm my right to grow and change," " I am grateful for my unique journey," or "I am moving toward achieving my goals."

Affirmations are supportive reminders of your efforts, achievements, and intentions. They are honest, strengths-based words of encouragement. They are the statements a caring, supportive person would say when standing next to you. Affirmations need not tell the entire story. For instance, an affirmation that focuses on self-approval would not mention the reality that you sometimes judge yourself. The point is to see your strengths.

Most of us devote plenty of time reminding ourselves of our deficits. Focusing on our strengths does not need to mean we are denying those deficits. We are simply choosing to direct our attention to the personal strengths and assets we possess. That's a healthy practice that can help us maintain our motivation to persevere through the struggles in life as we strive to achieve our goals.

Like mantras, the way you use an affirmation is entirely up to you. One method would be to set an intentional subject for a meditation by repeating a chosen affirmation three times: once prior to, once during, and once after a meditation. Repeating affirmations, whether during meditations or at other times, can help generate personal empowerment. In this way we can project a different kind of energy out into the world, creating opportunities for success for ourselves and for the people we touch.

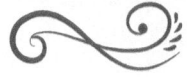

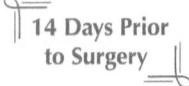

**14 Days Prior
to Surgery**

Fear

To be blind is not miserable;
not to be able to bear blindness, that is miserable.

— *John Milton*

We begin this meditative journey with fear. It's common for cosmetic patients to worry about a multitude of things. What will the doctor do to my appearance? Am I spending too much money? Will I have pain? Will the anesthesia be safe? Is this all a mistake?

Anxiety is normal, but too much of it is unhealthy. If you feel consumed by fearful thoughts, devote some time to using mindfulness practices to disengage from those thoughts. It's also helpful to confront the fears, to weaken their hold on you. Ask and answer these three questions to confront *any* fear at *any* time:

1. What is the likelihood that the feared thing will happen?

2. What is the likelihood I will be unable to *cope* with it, if it happens?

3. What steps can I take to prepare to cope if the feared thing happens?

Research suggests many of the things we worry about *never* happen. This is even more true if you tend to have high anxiety. So, use the exercise to reassure yourself.

> **Affirmations:** I affirm my ability to cope with whatever life sends me. I know that there is both joy and disappointment in life and I embrace that reality.
>
> **Mantras:** I can face my fears. I can cope.

**13 Days Prior
to Surgery**

Uncertainty

*Each time you stay present with fear and uncertainty, you're letting go of
a habitual way of finding security and comfort.*
— *Pema Chödrön*

Do you feel distressed at times because of uncertainty? Of course you do.
How could you not struggle with the reality of uncertainty at one time
or another? Surgical outcomes are not guaranteed. A patient and surgeon
might do all the right things, and yet the procedure might not produce
the expected outcome. Devote some meditations to sitting with this reality. This is what Pema Chödrön is referring to.

How else can you cope with uncertainty? First, clarify your thoughts
and confirm their accuracy. Second, "dose" yourself on thoughts that
focus on fears of unknowns. It's okay to allow yourself to think about
uncertainty—just don't do it too much.

You may need to schedule a specific time period for thinking about
concerns. Limit the time to thirty minutes or less, and only spend three to
four days a week on these thoughts. Once you designate the time:

1. Briefly note concerns as they occur to you during the day; and

2. Honor your self-promise to think about the concerns at the
   designated time.

   Affirmations: I embrace that uncertainty is part of my
   reality. I know that I have carefully planned for this
   procedure. I know that I have chosen a surgeon I trust and I
   act purposefully to achieve my goals.

   Mantras: I stay present. I accept all parts of my reality.

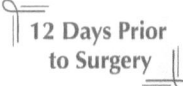

**12 Days Prior
to Surgery**

Pride

*Healthy pride is not arrogance. It is not a sense of superiority.
It is about acceptance, love, and nurturance of our entire self.*

— Alan Goodwin

Err on the side of too much self-affirmation rather than not enough. As you cope with reactions to your decision to undergo a cosmetic procedure, it's helpful to remember all the things you do and believe that are kind and well-intentioned. Take pride—in yourself.

Why do this now? Because people often punish themselves for choosing cosmetic work. Many cosmetic patients struggle with feelings of guilt or shame, sometimes internalizing criticisms without even being able to pinpoint the source.

How do *you* feel about yourself? That's what is important. Remind yourself of that. Take pride in who you are. Embrace a pride that is defined by self-acceptance, self-compassion, and gratitude. A pride that is self-affirming and self-protective.

Your body is *yours*. Only one person has the right to determine what will be done to it—YOU. Don't give that power away. It's yours.

> **Affirmations:** Today, I affirm myself. I know who I am and I know that I like myself. I affirm my inner strength and my dignity.

> **Mantras:** I feel proud. I affirm myself.

Positivity

*Sometimes in life we want to be the critic; to say what's wrong,
and how things should be. But sometimes, it's nice to take a break
and just enjoy the movie.*

— *Alan Goodwin*

You've decided to seek a cosmetic change. A courageous decision. You probably have several weeks before the procedure date. If it's already scheduled, you've signed pages of release forms. You know complications are possible, but not likely. Still, concerns and negative thoughts are hard to set aside. Why not devote today to the positive ones? Why not set aside some days to feel confident, eager, and grateful? How about today?

Engage in some good, healthy, refreshing image formation. Begin by setting aside the need to be strictly accurate. The future is never entirely predictable, so it's good to practice identifying positive possibilities? There's a time for strict accuracy. Allow today to *not* be one of those times.

Today, think or write about what you want to see when you look into the mirror in the future. Imagine how the surgery will change and improve your life. Envision the things you hope to encounter in other people. Write in as much detail as you can.

> **Affirmations:** Today, I affirm my right to be hopeful and eager. I give myself the gift of positivity. I affirm the power of my dreams to help me set goals that motivate me.

> **Mantras:** I embrace dreams. I embrace my future. I feel hopeful.

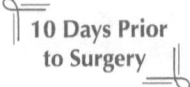
**10 Days Prior
to Surgery**

Fear: Anesthesia

To him who is in fear, everything rustles.
— Sophocles

Let's turn again to fears, because they can become destructive if not managed well. Our fear must be balanced. Fear protects us from harm, but too much fear is corrosive.

The quote from Sophocles reminds us of two truths: first, what we fear often does not even exist. And second, even when feared things do exist, we often don't accurately perceive them.

It's common for patients preparing for a surgical procedure to worry about the anesthesia. Patients sometimes worry they may not be anesthetized enough and will feel pain. Other patients worry they will receive too much anesthetic and will never awaken from the procedure.

If you are still worried about the anesthesia, or about any aspect of your planned procedure, gather accurate information about risks. Once you do this, make your decision about whether to move forward with the procedure. Once you decide to move forward, it's important to honor that decision and stop engaging the fears. For help disengaging from fears, use the mindfulness techniques in this book.

> **Affirmation:** Today I affirm that I have spoken with people about my fears and those people have reassured me.

> **Mantras:** I trust myself. I trust my doctors. I will be safe.

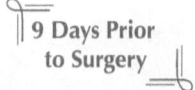
9 Days Prior to Surgery

Entitlement

"One recipe for happiness is to have a sense of entitlement."
To this she added a star, and noted at the bottom of the page:
"This is not a lesson I have ever been in a position to learn."

— Alan Bennett

Often, cosmetic surgery patients contact me to discuss entitlement. These clients typically struggle with a *lack* of entitlement. This problem is especially common in women. In many cultures, women learn from a young age that they should sacrifice their own needs for the benefit of others, particularly when the others are family members.

Cosmetic procedures are never inexpensive. Many clients have difficulty spending so much money on themselves. When my clients are struggling in this way, I sometimes take them through an uncomfortable exercise. I ask them to state the estimated cost of the procedure they are considering. I then ask them to name alternative ways they could spend that money. Answers have included:

1. A car for my son/daughter

2. One year of college tuition for my son/daughter

3. A boat for our family to use during the summer

4. One year of lodging for my elderly parent in a nicer facility

5. Dental work for my parent

6. New flooring for three rooms in my home

7. A new model airplane for my husband

8. A cosmetic procedure for my daughter

9. Sponsorship of my kid's soccer team

10. A dozen goats to be gifted to an indigent family in another nation

While exploring the many things the money could buy, we discuss the client's tendency to forgo their own needs in favor of worthy causes such as these. We discuss the idea that there will always be many worthwhile ways to spend money. Ultimately, the question becomes: at what point is it acceptable for you to do something just for *yourself*? Like most issues in psychotherapy, the value of the conversation lies more in the exploration of the subject than in finding a single correct answer.

One thing is clear: it's healthy to give ourselves gifts sometimes. We cannot nurture growth in others if we haven't nurtured it in ourselves. And, of course, we give loved ones an invaluable gift when we model self-care.

> **Affirmations:** Today, I affirm my right to care for my own needs, too.
>
> **Mantras:** I am entitled. It's okay to give to myself.

**8 Days Prior
to Surgery**

Reactions

Resolutely train yourself to attain peace.
— Buddha

As your surgery day nears, try to maintain a peaceful state of mind. A mind at peace is less likely to react with excess intensity, in either direction. It will be helpful to you if you commit to this. It's okay to be bothered by some things. It's just not good to be *too* bothered. When we are too bothered, we tend to create new discomfort—discomfort about the discomfort. A daily meditation practice can help you reduce these tendencies.

It is especially important to manage your reactions when you undergo a cosmetic procedure. Remember that your surgeon is like a skilled artist working with a canvas and medium that are, to some degree, unique. Begin now to embrace the work of art that will soon be created. Your happiness doesn't require that only good and expected things happen. It requires only that you accept events with grace and resiliency.

> **Affirmations:** Today, I affirm my ability to cope. I know that my mindset is the key to my ability to receive both the blessings and the challenges of life.

> **Mantras:** My mind is at peace. My thoughts are balanced. I am resilient.

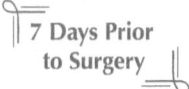

**7 Days Prior
to Surgery**

Second Thoughts

It is not the mountain we conquer, but ourselves.
— Sir Edmund Hillary

Your big day is drawing near. Having second thoughts? If not, devote today to celebrating that. Skip to the bottom of this page and read/use the affirmation and mantras.

If you *are* having second thoughts—STOP IT.

Did "STOP IT" work? No? Okay, let's explore this struggle together. At this late stage, second thoughts should not occur often, and they should be mild. You've considered your options and made your decisions. It's best now to honor those.

If your concerns persist and cause you to still consider cancelling the procedure, address them. Get accurate information. If necessary, call your doctor's office.

Persistent second thoughts are usually not because of information deficits. Typically, they reflect patterned ways some patients dishonor themselves and their decisions. If you know you have the tendency to do this to yourself, mindfulness practices can help you break the habit. Healthy distractions can also be healing because, as a form of self-care, they remind you that you deserve to be nurtured and respected.

> **Affirmation:** I know that this process confronts me with uncertainty, and I know that sometimes the uncertainty may cause me to sow doubt where none needs to exist.

> **Mantras:** I nurture my growth. I honor my decisions. I release my doubts.

Pain

Between stimulus and response there is a space.
In that space is our power to choose our response.
In our response lies our growth and our freedom.

— ***Viktor E. Frankl***

Do you worry about the pain you may feel during your recovery? I can't promise that you won't have discomfort—but I promise you can prepare for it.

First, ask questions. Ask your doctor and their staff to describe what you might feel and how you can cope—what lifestyle changes they recommend and medications they provide. You might ask how long the pain usually lasts and when it begins to subside. Remember that your experience might be different from the norm.

Next, prepare your healing space in whatever ways will bring you comfort. Have access to music, entertainment, or other healthy distractions. Make the space as comfortable for rest and healing as possible.

Beyond information, consider Frankl's words. Mindfulness and meditation address exactly what Frankl was talking about. You can prepare your mind to accept whatever comes. If you embrace the inevitability of occasional discomfort in life, you will tolerate it better. Meditation trains your mind to do that.

> **Affirmation:** Today, I affirm the reality of discomfort in life. I also affirm that I know that discomfort is temporary and that I can tolerate it.

> **Mantras:** I can cope. I am prepared.

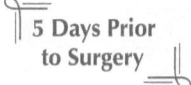

**5 Days Prior
to Surgery**

Beauty

*Most people acquire their definition of beauty
from other people. As if it were a gift
from a store that doesn't accept returns.*

— Alan Goodwin

How do you value beauty? How broad is your definition? Does it bring you comfort, or does it cause you to feel uneasy? Is it your own, or is it someone else's? Is it like a shirt that has never quite felt like it fit you?

Physical beauty is not supposed to matter so much. We are told "beauty is only skin-deep," and that we should not "judge a book by its cover." And yet we know that people notice the way we look. And so do we.

Particularly now, as your procedure date nears, is there anything you can do about this? There is. You can be mindful to choose a broad, affirming, and inclusive definition of beauty. There are many forms of physical beauty. You possess some of those. You also possess beauty that is not physical. Compassion, sense of humor, and generosity are a few examples of beautiful qualities. These or other beautiful qualities lie within you.

Today, commit to honoring all the parts of yourself that exhibit beauty.

> **Affirmation:** Today I affirm my desire to feel beautiful, and I also affirm that I am already beautiful in many ways. I affirm that my beauty resides within me, it is my essence, and that will never change.

> **Mantra:** I am beautiful—in many ways.

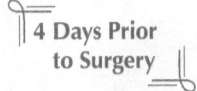

**4 Days Prior
to Surgery**

Self-Care

*This is a great cosmos, and you're a little cosmos within the great cosmos.
And, without you, the great cosmos is not complete.
So, appreciate the little cosmos.*

— Leo Buscaglia

Are you getting excited as you approach your procedure date? Are you envisioning and planning? Looking ahead to how you will grow and evolve with the help of this procedure? It's healthy and nurturing to give yourself the gift of intentions.

Another kind of preparation focuses on your recovery process. Knowing what helps you feel supported, and surrounding yourself with those people and things during your recovery, will nurture your healing.

Today, list the people and things you like to have near you when you need extra support. Some examples of what others have brought with them as they recover:

1. Close relatives or friends

2. Comfortable bedding

3. Music, audiobooks, movies, or other recorded entertainment

4. Healthy, doctor-recommended, convenient, prepared foods (Jell-O, rice, poached chicken, broth, hard-boiled eggs, bread, bananas, etc.)

5. Someone who can check sutures, drains, or bandages, as needed

6. Earplugs or eye masks for restful sleep, if doctor-permitted

7. Any object that brings you comfort

Affirmations: Today, I affirm that I am planning ahead. I know that I am preparing myself to have what I need during the healing process.

Mantra: I care for myself. I nurture my healing.

**3 Days Prior
to Surgery**

Critics

*When the snow oppresses the branches,
the pine tree nevertheless remains green.*

— *Japanese Proverb*

Have you told friends, relatives, or coworkers about your upcoming procedure? Were they supportive? When the people we care about seem unsupportive of important decisions, it can activate self-doubt. In some cases, clients feel deeply disappointed in those people.

It's very important to remember that many people are unable to respond based on *your* needs, values, and desires. Some of them respond based on what they believe *they* would do in your situation. Their responses are reflective of *their* struggle and *their* needs. It's best to resist the urge to assume that they intend to be unsupportive. Whatever their intentions, remember that there's no rule that you must have their approval. So, you really don't need to know why they were not more supportive.

Focus on yourself, not them. Nurture your empowerment. Prepare for your healing process. There will be plenty of time to discuss other peoples' intentions with them, after you have healed.

> **Affirmation:** Today, I affirm that I know what is best for me and I know that I am taking steps to achieve that.
>
> **Mantras:** I am strong. I know what I want. I support my growth.

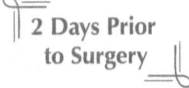

2 Days Prior to Surgery

Revolution

I believe the lasting revolution
comes from deep changes in ourselves
which influence our collective life.

— *Anaïs Nin*

You probably don't think of yourself as a revolutionary by virtue of your decision to undergo a cosmetic surgical procedure. But when we courageously seek voluntary change, we challenge the common tendency to allow the inertia of the status quo to prevent us from achieving growth and change.

Your surgical procedure represents a decision to assert your independence over your body. It represents your choice to venture out and make a change. And now, if you choose to, you can explore broader issues: how will personal change and revolution impact you? How might your changes inspire others to introduce changes into their lives? How do you envision modeling adjustment to change, as a way of supporting others in their processes of change and growth?

> **Affirmations:** Today, I affirm my role in a revolution—within myself. I affirm and embrace that my growth may even influence others.

> **Mantras:** I embrace change. I inspire others.

**1 Day Prior
to Surgery**

Grace

Ordinary women of grace are, in a sense, my real role models.
What always struck me is how unbitter they were.
They had the capacity to keep struggling.

— ***Marion Wright Edelman***

Life sends struggles our way. None of us is spared. One type of struggle is the recovery from a medical procedure. As you prepare for the procedure and your recovery, explore this question: *How do I respond to life's struggles?*

One response is grace. In religious contexts, grace is kindness granted to an undeserving sinner. For our purposes, we can think of grace as kindness informed by the recognition that we all struggle sometimes. In other words:

Grace = Kindness + Wisdom

This definition makes grace a close relative of compassion — the act of seeing all people — including yourself — within the context of their struggle.

See this compassionate form of grace within you. Choose to feel it. Allow it to fill you. Direct it toward yourself and others. In this way, grace will help you persevere through emotional and physical discomfort.

> **Affirmation:** Today, I affirm that I have an abundance of kindness and compassion within myself. I know that my inner strength is nurtured by grace.

> **Mantra:** I am filled with grace. I feel my compassion. I feel my wisdom.

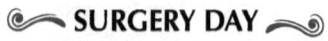

SURGERY DAY

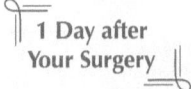
1 Day after Your Surgery

Achievements

Love yourself first and everything else falls into line.
— Lucille Ball

You did it. YOU—DID—IT!!! How do you feel about that? Did you wake up today feeling proud? If not, give that gift to yourself now. You have earned it. You made a major decision to do something important for yourself, and you followed through on it.

There will be time to feel other emotions, but today, allow yourself to lie back and appreciate yourself. You wanted something, and you persevered and got it. You gave yourself a job and you completed it. Great job!

> **Affirmations:** Today, I commit to seeing my strengths. I have evolved into a compassionate, resilient adult.

> **Mantras:** I can rely on myself. I feel proud of myself.

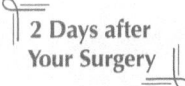

**2 Days after
Your Surgery**

Rest

*The secret of health for both mind and body is not to mourn for the past,
worry about the future, or anticipate troubles,
but to live in the present moment wisely and earnestly.*

— Buddha

Are you sleeping well? Sleep is necessary while healing. Sometimes worry interrupts our sleep. If your mind is active with worries while trying to sleep, try this exercise:

1. Keep a pad of paper and a pen next to your bed.

2. Write down any worry or thought you want to think more about.

3. Note in your mind that you need not "hold on to" that thought. It exists on paper. It will not disappear. You will think about it later.

4. Schedule a time the next day to think about the items on the paper.

This is a way to manage your thoughts. You get to decide when you do the "work" of planning and worrying. There are some times when it is best for your mind to rest and focus only on healing. This is one of those times.

> **Affirmations:** My concerns can wait until tomorrow. I care about myself and my body. I know that I can bring my body peace and rest.

> **Mantras:** I give my body rest. I will sleep soundly. I am at peace.

**3 Days after
Your Surgery**

Healing and Self-Care

The wound is the place where the light enters you.

— Rumi

Your body knows when it has been altered. It reacts to changes. It has had two days to adjust after the procedure. You have instructions from your doctor that tell you how to help your body heal at this time. Today is a good day to reaffirm your commitment—to your body. To your healing and recovery.

Have you checked your body in the ways your doctor suggested? If you are having difficulty doing that, have you enabled someone to help you? This is an important time. You have the opportunity to give your body the chance to create an outcome that fits with what you hoped to see.

Remember that swelling and bruising are common aspects of healing. If you have concerns, call your doctor. Get the reassurance you need to maintain a calm and reassured mindset while you continue to recover.

> **Affirmation:** Today, I affirm my commitment to my
> healing and recovery process. On this day I honor my body.
> I commit to healing and recovery.
>
> **Mantra:** I honor my body. I nurture my recovery. I am
> healing.

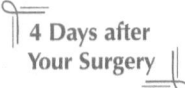

4 Days after Your Surgery

Resilience

Do not judge me by my success,
judge me by how many times I fell down and got back up again.
— Nelson Mandela

Has your resilience been tested? Resilience is often linked to the notion of immunity from weakness or exhaustion, or even from physical injury. But resilience isn't immunity from any of those. On the contrary, resilience can only exist within the context of struggle. We exhibit resilience when we show that we can bend without breaking. We can feel pain yet recognize it is temporary. We can cope and we can recover.

How resilient are you? When you don't get what you seek, how do you respond? How do you accept? How do you recover—and why?

As the results of your cosmetic procedure become clearer, you will have an opportunity to cope with an outcome. And that will be an opportunity to show yourself how well you can cope with whatever comes in life. Try to notice your process. And notice how you are treating yourself.

I promise you this: If you commit to being kind to yourself and to other people, you will have more contact with your resilient inner core. You have kindness to give to yourself and to others. Empower yourself by giving freely and often.

> **Affirmation:** Today I remember the strength within myself and I show it to myself through self-care.

> **Mantras:** I am strong. I am resilient. I am kind.

Solitude

Solitude is like punctuation. A paragraph without periods and commas would be exhausting to read.

— *Arnie Kozak*

Healing processes impose some periods of solitude. Sometimes it feels good to be alone. At other times, the healing process can activate feelings of loneliness. Discomfort leads some people to seek the company of others, whereas it leads others to seek solitude.

Allow yourself to find a balance between aloneness and togetherness. While healing, it's good to have time to connect with yourself. It helps you get in touch with your body. It's also helpful to set aside time to devote your healing resources to yourself.

But too much solitude can be unhealthy. When others are present, we get to feel cared for, but we also get to care for others, which can aid healing. If you are alone, you may want to reach out to others with a phone call, a text message, or a message on social media. When you feel up to it, meet someone for a coffee or a walk in a park.

> **Affirmation:** Today I affirm my value for the relationships I have in my life, including my relationship with myself. I honor them, and myself, by nurturing them.

> **Mantra:** I value togetherness. I value time with myself. I am never alone.

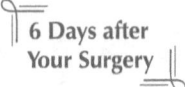

Disillusionment

*Better to allow mirrors to suffer
from disuse than misuse.*
— **Alan Goodwin**

Have you had one of those days lately? A day when you look into the mirror, over and over, concerned, maybe even disillusioned?

Excessive use of mirrors is never healthy, but it's particularly unhelpful during this healing phase. It dishonors your decision to have had the procedure, and it often fuels self-abuse. It's healthy to look, now and again, but not too much. If you can't help yourself, it may be best to stop altogether. See if you can find someone to whom to delegate all healing monitoring. Use mindfulness exercises to try to help yourself reduce or stop looking. And leave as much of the looking as possible to when you see your physician for the postoperative checkups.

> **Affirmation:** Today I remember how important it is for me to honor my past decisions and to treat myself with dignity, love, and respect.

> **Mantra:** I honor myself. I honor my decisions.

**7 Days after
Your Surgery**

Gratitude

Gratitude is a vision correction tool.
Without gratitude, we see either the forest or the trees.
With gratitude, we see both.

— Alan Goodwin

Do you value your own mind? Does that sound like a strange idea? After all, your mind helped you assess your options, choose a surgical procedure, and select a physician. Can you appreciate the abilities that enabled you to do those things? Or do you insist on minimizing your role, attributing your decisions to friends or family members who supported you? Or to the physician?

Here's the truth: *you* made those decisions. Honor that today. Allow yourself to honor your mind and your commitment to take action for yourself. Recognize that you have been blessed with a mind capable of making complex decisions. Devote today to feeling grateful not only for the love and support in your life, but also for your ability to think through your options and act decisively.

> **Affirmations:** I know that my life is improved because of the mind I have been blessed with. Today, I affirm that my mind has brought gifts into my life.

> **Mantras:** My mind is strong and healthy. I feel blessed.

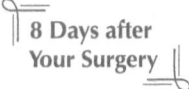

8 Days after Your Surgery

Mindfulness

Life is like that. We don't know anything.
We call something bad; we call it good.
But really, we just don't know.

— **Pema Chödrön**

There is much you don't know right now. You may still have bandages. You may have swelling or bruising. You may have soreness. You may be feeling withdrawn and irritable. Healing is a difficult, sometimes scary process.

Mindfulness practices and meditation help us maintain a healthy mindset. Our thoughts can become predatory. Meditation can help us detach from unhealthy thoughts.

If you are struggling with fearful thoughts, try to structure your day such as by scheduling when you will complete the tasks that your doctor gave you. Focus on mindfulness practices such as meditation and healthy distractions. These can help you avoid compulsively engaging in unhealthy habits such as excessive self-monitoring, worrying, or eating. Simplify things. Your job now is just to recover.

> **Affirmations:** On this day I remember that my trust in the process is a gift I possess. I choose to trust my doctor, the procedure, and the healing journey.

> **Mantra:** I trust the process. Healing is a journey.

**9 Days after
Your Surgery**

Risk—and Courage

*Why not go out on a limb?
That's where the fruit is.*

— Will Rogers

Will Rogers knew it, and now you do, too: some of the ripest fruit life has to offer hangs on the tips of branches, far away from the trunk, near the tops of trees. You have climbed and climbed, and slid along branches, high above the ground, to reach the fruit. You are almost there.

There are still some days of recovery before your end result can be known. Why not devote today to savoring the view from the tree tops? Appreciate that you have brought yourself to this point. You've walked a winding path. A long path that requires commitment and stamina. And you have been strong. You will reach the fruit soon.

> **Affirmation:** Today, I honor that my willingness to take risks has brought me to this place. I affirm that I chose this path, knowing the destination is uncertain and I am eager to I honor my willingness to take risks.

> **Mantra:** I honor my courage. I embrace uncertainty.

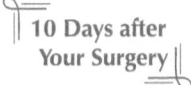
10 Days after Your Surgery

Faith

Stand straight, walk proud, have a little faith.
— **Garth Brooks**

Some things in life are not certain, like the outcome of a cosmetic procedure. Until you have completely healed, you can't know exactly how you will look. Sometimes this takes months of waiting. Tolerating months of uncertainty is a tall order. The coping tools in this book can help you. I hope they do.

There is one method of coping with uncertainty that we have not yet discussed: faith. The power of faith is that it leaves plenty of room for acceptance of both the blessings and the challenges of life. A peaceful coexistence with both is the goal of mindfulness. This is why a core principle underlying mindfulness practices is this:

The most powerful force undermining our ability
to cope with the struggles of life
is our rejection of the struggles.

So, as opposed to denying the struggles, or resisting them, we can choose to focus on our faith that we can cope with them. You can choose to have faith in your doctors and in your body and your mind.

> **Affirmations:** On this day, I commit to living in faith. I commit to being present authentically and to remaining faithful.

> **Mantras:** Uncertainty is temporary. Faith is permanent.

Secrets

One person's secrecy is another person's privacy.
— *Alan Goodwin*

Keeping secrets is considered good when they are entrusted to us, but when the secret is our own, we sometimes feel pressured to disclose it. We are made to feel dishonest if we keep it. Sometimes people don't feel safe sharing particular information with certain people. When those people are close friends or relatives, it creates an unpleasant dilemma.

Have you chosen *not* to tell some people about your cosmetic procedure? How do you feel about that? The age of social media has caused a blurring of the line between public and private. Many people seem to have no line and they often urge that we all should live that way.

If you feel dishonest for not telling everyone about your procedure, give yourself the gift of thinking of it as private information rather than as a secret. We disclose private information only if the nature of the relationship warrants it. Private information is often simply not relevant to certain relationships. Shouldn't you get to decide this?

> **Affirmations:** Today, I affirm that I own my personal health information. I may choose to share elements of it with others—or not.
>
> **Mantras:** I'm entitled to privacy. It's okay to protect myself.

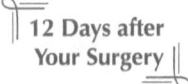

**12 Days after
Your Surgery**

Regrets

*Many of us crucify ourselves between two thieves,
regret for the past and fear of the future.*
— Fulton Oursler

Are you feeling regret? *Uh oh.* It's less than two weeks after the procedure. It's too soon for that. There is so much you don't yet know about the eventual outcome. And once you see it, you will need to give yourself enough of a chance to adjust to it.

First, be very clear about your concerns. Once you identify a concern, ask yourself: do I have accurate information about the source of my feelings of regret?

Sometimes we feel regrets or worries for reasons unrelated to whatever is truly happening. For instance, troubling thoughts distract us from other pain. They are often smoke screens, covering up something else going on within us. Instead of focusing on the worries, it's better to focus on maintaining your healthy recovery. Eat well, get rest, and do the things your doctor told you to do.

If you still feel the need to focus on regrets, do it in writing for a scheduled and limited time today. Limit how much energy you devote to regrets. It's not constructive to think a lot about them until after your healing and recovery process is complete. And then only if there is something to truly regret.

> **Affirmation:** I honor my decision to undergo a procedure by focusing on my healing and recovery until they are complete.

> **Mantras:** I nurture my healing. All in good time.

**13 Days after
Your Surgery**

Kindness

Without light, nothing flowers.
— *May Sarton*

You are in that strange period: the procedure is done, but you await "the reveal." You may still wear bandages. You likely have swelling, discoloration, sensitivity, numbness, or other challenges. You are healing.

You must continue to get plenty of rest and care for yourself. One way to do that is sit or recline in a position that allows you to completely relax all of your muscles. Allow your body to heal. Some people like to listen to a loving kindness meditation as they imagine being filled with healing light and calming warmth. You could also listen to comforting music while quietly and slowly repeating a mantra.

Remember that we show kindness to ourselves when we remind ourselves of the sources of gratitude in our lives. The feeling of sunshine on your face. The sound of rain. Observing the spectacular beauty in nature, whether in a tiny plant or a glorious mountain. Be kind to yourself by soaking in your gratitude.

> **Affirmation:** Today, I affirm my commitment to the entire healing process.

> **Mantras:** I treat myself with kindness. I nurture my healing. I am healing.

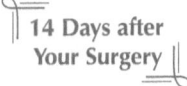

14 Days after Your Surgery

Presence

Life can be found only in the present moment.
The past is gone, the future is not yet here,
And if we do not go back to ourselves in the present moment
We cannot be in touch with life.

— *Thich Nhat Hanh*

Life is a series of moments. In one moment we feel confident in our direction and in who we are. At other times, we feel less certain, less clear in our thoughts. Our minds can feel like storm cells, our thoughts churning, generating thunder, lightning, torrential rains, and violent wind gusts. At those times, you may feel aimless. Or, you may fear you are moving toward somewhere you don't want to go.

But...trust. Persist. If you persist, things will become clear again. The sun in your mind will return. You are on your path. Even on days when it doesn't seem like it, you are progressing. This is your unique journey. Embrace it. Even when you feel lost, stay. Remain present. Observe. Be. One moment at a time.

> **Affirmations:** With every moment, I know I am closer to finding inner peace. I affirm that finding peace sometimes comes only after a struggle.

> **Mantras:** I stay present. One moment at a time.

APPENDIX A:

Other Resources for Readers

Cosmetic Procedures

1. *The Essential Cosmetic Surgery Companion.* Robert Kotler, MD.

2. *The Smart Woman's Guide to Plastic Surgery.* Jean Loftus, MD.

3. *Straight Talk about Cosmetic Surgery.* Arthur Perry, MD.

4. *Navigate Your Beauty: Smart and Safe Plastic Surgery Solutions.* Rod Rohrich, MD.

5. *Look Younger Now: Fillers, Face Lifts and Everything in Between - a 21st Century Guide.* Patrick Flaharty, MD.

6. *The Cosmetic Surgery Companion: A Consumer's Guide to the Latest Surgical Techniques to Improve Your Body from Head to Toe.* Antonia Mariconda.

7. *Your Beauty Advocate: A No-Nonsense Guide to Age-Defying Skincare Products and Procedures.* Kristy Hall.

8. *The Park Avenue Face: Secrets and Tips from a Top Facial Plastic Surgeon for Flawless, Undetectable Procedures and Treatments.* Andrew Jacono, MD.

9. *Killer Breasts: Overcoming Breast Implant Illness: A Compassionate Step-by-Step Guide to Cleanse Your Body, Heal Your Hormones and Ignite Your Life.* Diane Kazer, FDN.

10. *Your Survival Guide to Cosmetic Surgery.* Anthony LaBruna, MD.

11. *After the Cut: How to Prepare For and Recover From Cosmetic Plastic Surgery.* Nicole Psomas, PT, MS.

12. *Botox: The Truth About Botox Injections: An Introductory Guide to Botulinum Toxin Procedures, Costs, Options, And What You Must Know.* Arnold Hendrix.

13. *Botox and Beyond: Your Guide To Safe, Nonsurgical, Cosmetic Procedures.* Jerome Potozkin, MD.

14. *Plastic Surgery Recovery Handbook.* Kathleen Helen Lisson, CLT.

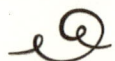

Body Image

1. *Reshaping the Female Body: The Dilemma of Cosmetic Surgery.* Kathy Davis.

2. *The Body Image Workbook 2nd Edition: An Eight-Step Program for Learning to Like Your Looks.* Thomas F. Cash, PhD.

3. *Feeling Good about the Way You Look: A Program for Overcoming Body Image Problems.* Sabine Wilhelm, PhD. New York: Guilford Press.

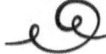

Mindfulness

1. *The Mindfulness Solution.* Ronald Siegel, Psy.D.

2. *Good Medicine.* Pema Chödron.

3. *Body and Mind Are One.* Thich Nhat Hanh.

4. *Mindfulness in Plain English.* Bhante Gunaratana.

APPENDIX B:

List of Tools

Journal Exercises:

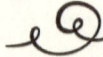

Screening Tools:

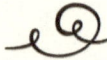

Meditations:

ABOUT THE AUTHOR

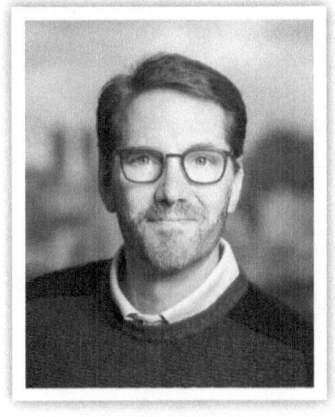

Dr. Alan Goodwin is a licensed psychologist, public speaker, educator, and author. Based in Los Angeles, he has devoted the past 22 years to developing a form of Mindfulness-based Cognitive-Behavioral Psychotherapy that is active, educational, and affirming of his clients' innate strengths and abilities to grow and change. His goal-directed method involves a blending of warmth, humor, and assertiveness. All of these qualities are on full display in *Saving Face Without Losing Your Mind: Bringing Mindfulness to Your Cosmetic Procedure.* You can find more of his informational videos, meditations, and self-help tools at DrAlanGoodwin.com.